Dedication

In memory of Gordon Hartman (1936–2004), friend and colleague whose enthusiasm and encyclopaedic knowledge were an asset to all who knew him.

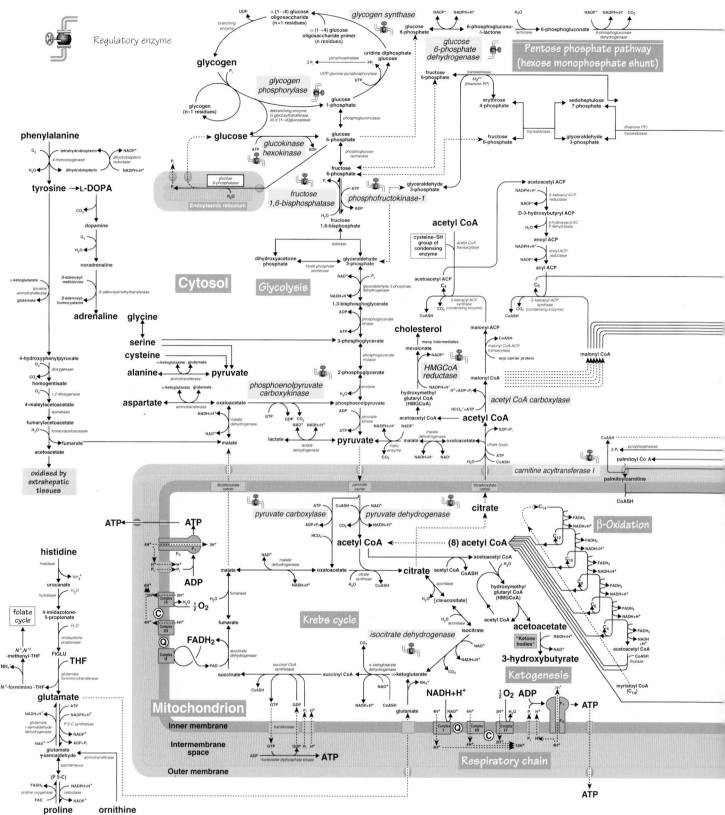

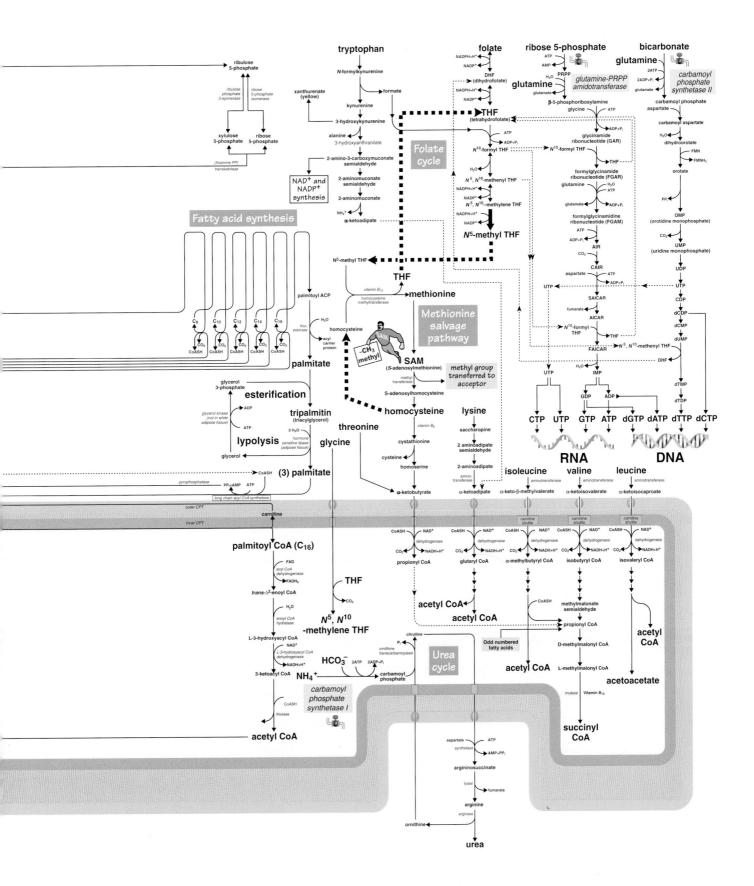

Medical Biochemistry at a Glance

Medical Biochemistry at a Glance

Dr J. G. Salway

School of Biomedical and Molecular Sciences
University of Surrey
Guildford
Surrey, UK

Third edition

A John Wiley & Sons, Ltd., Publication

First edition published 1996
Second edition published 2006
Second edition translations:
Chinese Translation 2007 Taiwan Yi Hsien Publishing Co. Ltd
Japanese Translation 2007 Medical Sciences International Ltd, Tokyo
Korean Translation 2007 E*PUBLIC KOREA Co. Ltd
Polish Translation 2009 Górnicki Wydawnictwo Medyczne

Library of Congress Cataloging-in-Publication Data
Salway, J. G.
   Medical biochemistry at a glance. – 3rd ed. / J.G. Salway.
        p. ; cm. – (At a glance)
   Includes bibliographical references and index.
   ISBN-13: 978-0-470-65451-4 (pbk. : alk. paper)
   ISBN-10: 0-470-65451-1 (pbk. : alk. paper)   1. Biochemistry–Outlines, syllabi, etc.   2. Clinical biochemistry–Outlines, syllabi, etc.   I. Title.   II. Series: At a glance series (Oxford, England)
   [DNLM: 1. Biochemical Phenomena.   QU 34]
   QP514.2.G76 2012
   612'.015–dc23
                                    2011024248

A catalogue record for this book is available from the British Library.

Set in 9 on 11.5 pt Times by Toppan Best-set Premedia Limited
Printed and bound in Singapore by Markono Print Media Pte Ltd

3   2017

Contents

Companion website

This book is accompanied by a companion website which contains interactive Multiple-Choice Questions:

www.ataglanceseries.com/medicalbiochemistry

Preface to the third edition

The subject matter in *Medical Biochemistry at a Glance* is selected from the biochemistry content of *First Aid for the USMLE Step 1*: the most popular guide used by students preparing for examinations. As such, it is written for medical students, but is equally accessible to students of the biomedical sciences such as biochemists, medical laboratory scientists, veterinary scientists, dentists, pharmacologists, physiologists, physiotherapists, nutritionists, food scientists, nurses, medical physicists, microbiologists and students of sports science. This book aspires to present medical biochemistry in the concise two-page format of the "At a Glance" series.

Students who study biochemistry as a subsidiary part of their course are frequently overwhelmed by the complexity and huge amount of detail involved. Lecturers will be familiar with the anxious expression of students as they complain "*How much of this do we need to know?*" or "*Do we need to memorise all the structural formulae and the chemical reactions?*" In fairness, biochemistry **is** a complex and heavily detailed subject. Students should have two objectives: (i) **to study** and **understand** biochemical concepts and reactions but **not necessarily memorise** the structural details, (ii) **to prepare for examinations** by

determining the amount of detail required by intelligent perusal of lecture notes and past examination papers.

Medical Biochemistry at a Glance is written with these two objectives in mind. Judicious study of the back inside cover featuring a metabolic chart including formulae and the enzymes catalysing the reactions plus the comprehensive chart on the front inside cover will enable an understanding of metabolic biochemistry. The enzymes which regulate metabolic pathways are indicated in both charts and throughout the book. In the text of the book, complex detail is subjugated to a faint background so as to emphasise the most important aspects of the topic. However, students must familiarise themselves with the requirements of their particular examination board to determine how much should be trusted to memory.

Finally, the inspiration for *Medical Biochemistry at a Glance* has developed from my book *Metabolism at a Glance*. The latter is a more advanced book but the similarity of style between these two books facilitates progression to a higher level by students specialising in metabolism and disorders of metabolism.

Acknowledgements to the third edition

Following discussion with my editor, it was clear this new, third edition must include a section on "Molecular Biology": not my strongest subject. So the start of this book was marked by a four-day trip to Cheshire visiting my friends Dr Peter Barth and his wife Jane. Peter has dedicated his career to molecular biology and so I was most fortunate when he offered to update me in this fascinating subject. Jane provided excellent food and warm hospitality in their beautiful house. Peter's patient, clear and authoritative tuition defined the structure of the chapters. We also made time for recreation, and together they gave me a most enjoyable, productive and unforgettable visit. Peter's support, advice and encouragement continued through to the last moments of the final proofs. This book would not have been possible without Peter's invaluable help.

Once again I have been very fortunate to work with Elaine Leggett of Oxford Designers & Illustrators and the facilities provided by Mr Richard Corfield and his team. Elaine's first task was to update the artwork colour scheme from the second edition to full colour. Then, with her customary aplomb and talent she rose to the challenge of interpreting my sketches for the new Molecular Biology section.

At a Christmas drinks party, I met my old colleague Professor Peter Goldfarb. Inspired with Yuletide spirit, he offered help and generously gave his time, wise advice with characteristic attention to detail and constructive criticism.

I am very grateful to readers who have emailed to report errors and to friends and colleagues for expert advice, especially Dr Kimberly Dawdy, Dr Lucy Elphick, Dr Anna Gloyn, Professor Keith Frayn, Mrs

Rosemary James, Professor Gary John, Professor George Kass, Dr Lisa Meira, and Dr Helen Stokes.

Also, I wish again to record my gratitude to those who contributed to the second edition of this book, namely: Professor Loranne Agius, Dr Wynne Aherne, Dr Beatrice Evans, Dr Martyn Egerton, Professor George Elder, Dr Janet Brown, Dr Geoffrey Gibbons, Dr Barry Gould, Dr Bruce Griffin, Professor Stephen Halloran, Professor Chris O'Callaghan, Dr Anna Saada, and Mrs Marie Skerry.

Many reviewers commented on the excellent index compiled by Philip Aslett for the second edition, so I was very pleased when he agreed to help once more.

My editor Martin Davies has been exceptionally supportive. He has replied to my emails with extraordinary promptness and provided every facility requested to ensure efficient completion of the work. Also, it has been a great pleasure to work with other members of a most professional Wiley-Blackwell team, especially Heather Addison, Lesley Aslett, Helen Harvey, Karen Moore, Laura Murphy, and Beth Norton.

Regrettably, omissions and errors will have occurred and I would be most grateful to have these drawn to my attention.

Finally, I am grateful to my wife Nicky once again for her support, and for tolerating the intrusion of publication deadlines into our social programme; also the accumulation of documents and papers associated with writing this book.

J. G. Salway
Surrey, UK
j.salway@btinternet.com

Figure key

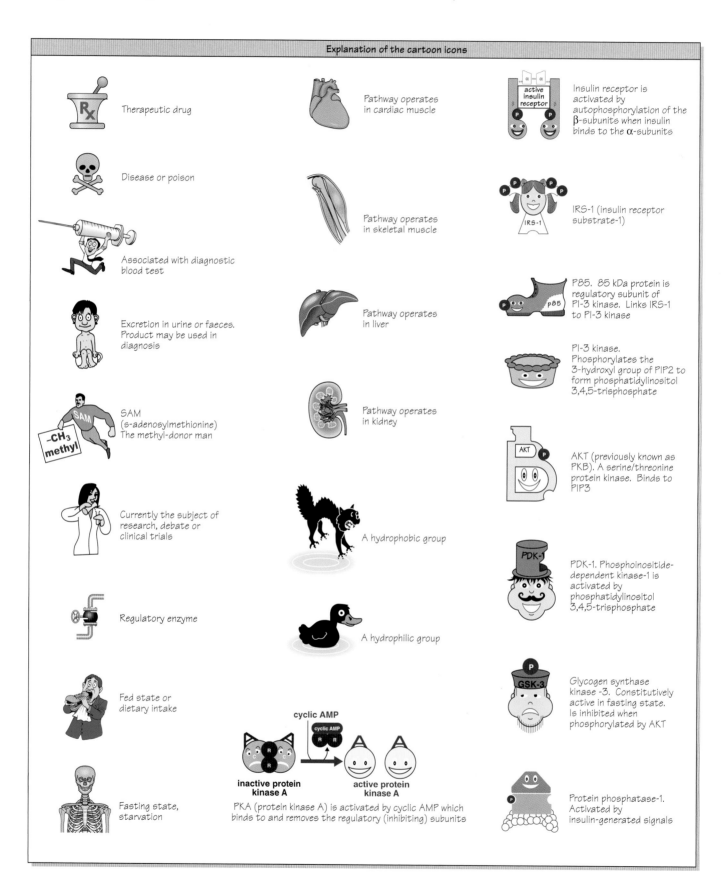

Explanation of the cartoon icons

Therapeutic drug

Disease or poison

Associated with diagnostic blood test

Excretion in urine or faeces. Product may be used in diagnosis

SAM (s-adenosylmethionine) The methyl-donor man

Currently the subject of research, debate or clinical trials

Regulatory enzyme

Fed state or dietary intake

Fasting state, starvation

Pathway operates in cardiac muscle

Pathway operates in skeletal muscle

Pathway operates in liver

Pathway operates in kidney

A hydrophobic group

A hydrophilic group

cyclic AMP

inactive protein kinase A

active protein kinase A

PKA (protein kinase A) is activated by cyclic AMP which binds to and removes the regulatory (inhibiting) subunits

Insulin receptor is activated by autophosphorylation of the β-subunits when insulin binds to the α-subunits

IRS-1 (insulin receptor substrate-1)

P85. 85 kDa protein is regulatory subunit of PI-3 kinase. Links IRS-1 to PI-3 kinase

PI-3 kinase. Phosphorylates the 3-hydroxyl group of PIP2 to form phosphatidylinositol 3,4,5-trisphosphate

AKT (previously known as PKB). A serine/threonine protein kinase. Binds to PIP3

PDK-1. Phosphoinositide-dependent kinase-1 is activated by phosphatidylinositol 3,4,5-trisphosphate

Glycogen synthase kinase -3. Constitutively active in fasting state. Is inhibited when phosphorylated by AKT

Protein phosphatase-1. Activated by insulin-generated signals

SI/mass unit conversions

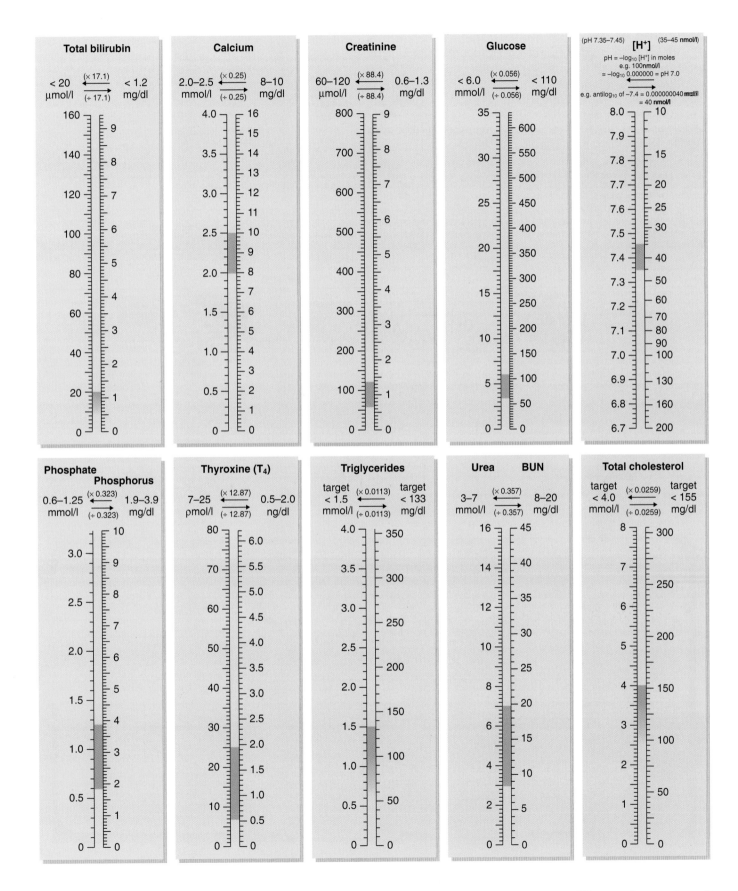

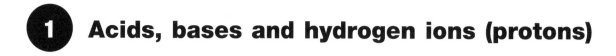

1 Acids, bases and hydrogen ions (protons)

Definition of pH

pH is defined as "*the negative logarithm to the base 10 of the hydrogen ion concentration*",

$$pH = -\log_{10}[H^+]$$

For example, at pH 7.0, the hydrogen ion concentration is $0.000\,000\,1$ mmoles/litre or 10^{-7} mmol/l.

The $\log_{10}$ of 0.0000001 is -7.0

Therefore, the negative $\log_{10}$ is $-(-7.0)$, i.e. $+7.0$ and hence the pH is 7.0.

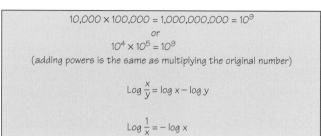

$$10,000 \times 100,000 = 1,000,000,000 = 10^9$$
$$or$$
$$10^4 \times 10^5 = 10^9$$
(adding powers is the same as multiplying the original number)

$$\text{Log } \frac{x}{y} = \log x - \log y$$

$$\text{Log } \frac{1}{x} = -\log x$$

Figure 1.1 Revision of logarithms.

Number	Equivalent as 10 to the power "n"	Logarithm$_{10}$
1000	10^3	3.0
100	10^2	2.0
10	10^1	1.0
1	10^0	0
0.1	10^{-1}	-1.0
0.01	10^{-2}	-2.0
$0.000\,000\,1$	10^{-7}	-7.0

Figure 1.2 Examples of numbers and their logarithms.

Number	Logarithm$_{10}$
1	0
2	0.301
3	0.477
4	0.602
5	0.699
6	0.778
7	0.845
8	0.903
9	0.954
10	1.0
20	1.301
30	1.477
200	2.301
2000	3.301

Units	Alternative representation
1 Mole per litre	1 mol/l
0.001 Mole per litre	1 mmol/l
0.000 001 Mole per litre	1 μmol/l
0.000 000 001 Mole per litre	1 nmol/l

Figure 1.3 Understanding units.

pH value	Equivalent in other concentration units
pH 1	0.1 Moles hydrogen ions/litre, or
	10^{-1} Moles hydrogen ions/litre, or
	10^{-1} g hydrogen ions per litre
pH 14	0.000 000 000 000 01 Moles/litre, or
	10^{-14} Moles hydrogen ions/litre, or
	10^{-14} g hydrogen ions /litre

Figure 1.5 pH and equivalent values.

Definition of a base:
A base is a substance that accepts a proton (i.e. a hydrogen ion, H^+) to form an acid, e.g. lactate is a conjugate base that accepts a proton to form lactic acid
Definition of an acid:
An acid is a compound that dissociates in water to release a proton (i.e. a hydrogen ion, H^+), e.g. lactic acid
A strong acid
(e.g. hydrochloric acid) is one that readily dissociates in water to release a proton.
A weak acid
(e.g. uric acid) is one that does not readily dissociate in water (e.g. to form urate and a proton)

Figure 1.4 Brønsted and Lowry definition of acids and bases.

Acidotic arterial blood pH values		Clinical examples
pH 6.8	160 nmol/l	
pH 6.9	130 nmol/l	metabolic acidosis, e.g. diabetic ketoacidosis, renal tubular acidosis
pH 7.0	100 nmol/l	
pH 7.1	80 nmol/l	
pH 7.2	63 nmol/l	respiratory acidosis
pH 7.3	50 nmol/l	
Normal arterial blood pH values		
pH 7.35	45 nmol/l	
pH 7.36	44 nmol/l	normal arterial blood pH
pH 7.38	42 nmol/l	
pH 7.40	40 nmol/l	pH range is 7.35 to 7.45 (45 to 35 nMoles H⁺/litre)
pH 7.42	38 nmol/l	
pH 7.44	36 nmol/l	
pH 7.45	35 nmol/l	
Alkalotic arterial blood pH values		Clinical examples
pH 7.5	32 nmol/l	
pH 7.6	26 nmol/l	
pH 7.7	20 nmol/l	metabolic alkalosis
pH 7.8	16 nmol/l	respiratory alkalosis
pH 7.9	13 nmol/l	
pH 8.0	10 nmol/l	

Figure 1.6 Examples of pH values seen in clinical practice.

What is pH?

pH is "the "power of hydrogen". It represents "the negative logarithm$_{10}$ of the hydrogen ion concentration". So why make things so complicated: why not use the plain and simple "hydrogen ion concentration"? Well, the concept was invented by a chemist for chemists and has advantages in chemistry laboratories. In clinical practice we are concerned with arterial values between pH 6.9 and 7.9. However, chemists need to span the entire range of pH values from pH 1 to pH 14. Values in terms of pH enable a convenient compression of numbers compared with the alternative which would be extremely wide-ranging as shown in Fig. 1.3. Figure 1.6 shows the normal reference range for pH in blood and, *in extremis*, fatal ranges that may be seen in acidotic or alkalotic diseases.

The pH scale is not linear

"The patient's blood pH has changed by 0.3 pH unit" **means it has doubled (or halved) in value.**

It is sometimes stated that "the patient's arterial blood pH has increased/decreased by, for example, 0.2 pH unit". However, notice that because of the logarithmic scale, this can misrepresent the true change in traditional concentration units. For example, a fall of 0.2 pH units from pH 7.20 to pH 7.00 represents 37 nmol/l, whereas a decrease from pH 7.00 to pH 6.8 represents a change of 60 nmol/l.

Also note that because the $\log_{10}$ of 2 = 0.3 (that is $2 = 10^{0.3}$), a decrease in pH by 0.3, e.g. from pH 7.40 to pH 7.10, represents a two-fold increase in H⁺ concentration, i.e. from 40 nmol/l to 80 nmol/l.

Similarly, an increase in pH from pH 7.40 to pH 7.70 represents a fall in H⁺ concentration from 40 nmol/l to 20 nmol/l.

The Henderson–Hasselbalch equation

A weak acid dissociates as shown:

$$HB \quad \rightleftharpoons \quad H^+ \quad + \quad B^-$$
$$\text{weak acid} \qquad \text{proton + conjugate base}$$

where **HB is the weak acid** that dissociates to a proton **H⁺** and its **conjugate base B⁻**. *NB Traditionally authors refer to the conjugate base as "A⁻"*, i.e. the initial letter of **a**cid, *which is perhaps confusing.*

Therefore from the Law of Mass Action where K = dissociation constant:

$$K = \frac{[H^+] + [B^-]}{[HB]}$$

Taking logs:

$$\log K = \log[H^+] + \log[B^-] - \log[HB]$$
$$\therefore -\log[H^+] = -\log K + \log[B^-] - \log[HB]$$
$$\text{i.e. } pH = pK + \log\frac{[B^-]}{[HB]}$$

Hence the Henderson–Hasselbalch equation:

$$pH = pK + \log\frac{[\text{conjugate base}]}{[\text{acid}]}$$

Clinical relevance of the Henderson–Hasselbalch equation

This is illustrated by respiratory acidosis and respiratory alkalosis. **The equation shows that:**

$$pH = pK + \log\frac{[\text{conjugate base}]}{[\text{acid}]}$$

Therefore in the case of the bicarbonate buffer system:

$$pH \propto \log\frac{[HCO_3^-]}{pCO_2}$$

Or, alternatively, the hydrogen ion concentration $[H^+] \propto \dfrac{pCO_2}{[HCO_3^-]}$.

In other words, the hydrogen ion concentration is proportional to the ratio of the amount of CO_2 to bicarbonate concentration in the blood. Hence, in **hypercapnia** (high blood CO_2 concentration) such as in respiratory acidosis, the ratio of pCO_2 to HCO_3^- is abnormally **high**, therefore the [H⁺] is **high** (i.e. pH is **low**).

Alternatively, **hypocapnia** caused by hyperventilation results in respiratory alkalosis. In this condition, **low** blood CO_2 concentrations prevail so the hydrogen ion concentration [H⁺] is **low** (i.e. pH is **high**).

The clinical relevance of pH and buffers will be described further in Chapters 2–5.

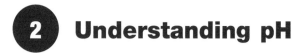

2 Understanding pH

Why do so many students have difficulty understanding acid/base theory?

The arcane jargon used in acid/base theory bewilders

Acid/base theory is often considered a difficult subject. It involves an understanding of acids and their ability to dissociate to form a conjugate base and hydrogen ions H⁺ (which are "protons"). As long ago as

1962 Creese *et al.* wrote in the *Lancet**: *"**There is a bewildering variety of pseudoscientific jargon in medical writing on this subject."** Difficulties arise because of this antiquated nomenclature, which is illustrated by the dialogue below:

*Creese R, Neil MW, Ledingham JM, Vere DW (1962) The terminology of acid–base regulation. *Lancet* **i**, 419.

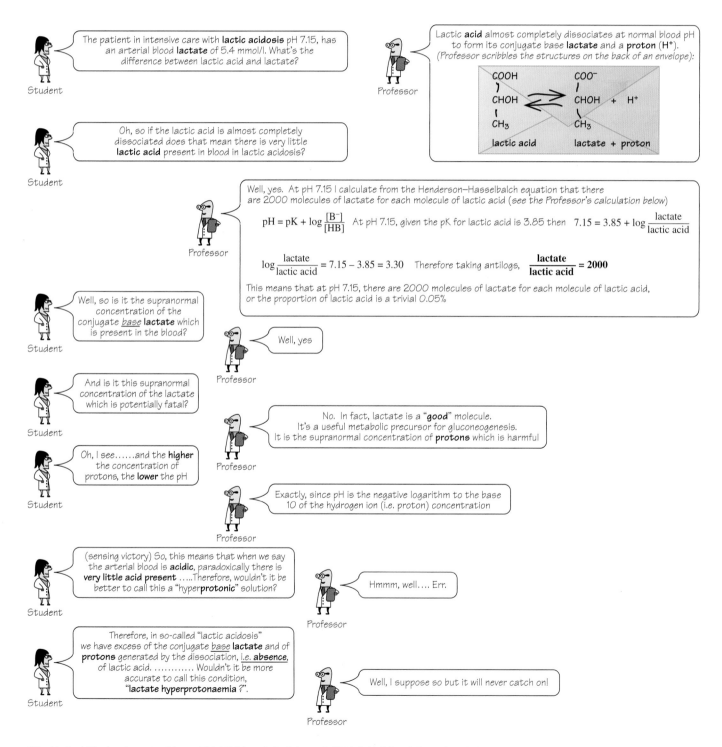

Dissociation of lactic acid

Figure 2.1 shows how the ratio of lactate : lactic acid varies with pH. When the proportion of lactate and lactic acid are identical (i.e. the ratio is 1), the pH equals the pK for lactic acid, i.e. the pK for lactic acid is 3.85.

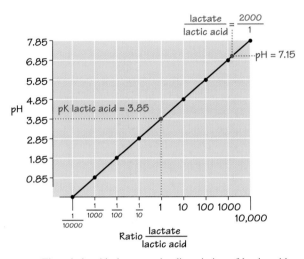

Figure 2.1 The relationship between the dissociation of lactic acid and pH, showing how the ratio of lactate : lactic acid varies with pH. When the proportion of lactate and lactic acid are identical (i.e. the ratio is 1), the pH equals the pK for lactic acid (i.e. the pK of lactic acid is 3.85).

Lactic acid and the bicarbonate buffer system

It takes only a few minutes to demonstrate this at home *in vivo*. Simply exercise anaerobically by running as fast as you can, preferably uphill, until you are breathless. In this time, through anaerobic glycolysis, your muscles will have generated **lactic acid** that dissociates to **lactate** and a **proton [H⁺]** (Fig. 2.2).† The protons must be removed and this is achieved when **bicarbonate** reacts with **[H⁺]** to form **carbonic acid**, which spontaneously breaks down to water and CO_2. The increased concentration of CO_2 stimulates the lungs to hyperventilate, thereby blowing off the excess CO_2 formed.

---

† The production of protons accompanying the formation of lactate shown in Fig. 2.2 is not strictly correct and has been fudged, just as it has been in (probably) all textbooks. Readers who are not satisfied with this traditional (but incorrect) explanation of proton production should read: Robergs RA, Ghiasvand F, Parker D (2004) Biochemistry of exercise-induced metabolic acidosis. *Am J Physiol Regul Integr Comp Physiol* **287**, R502–16.

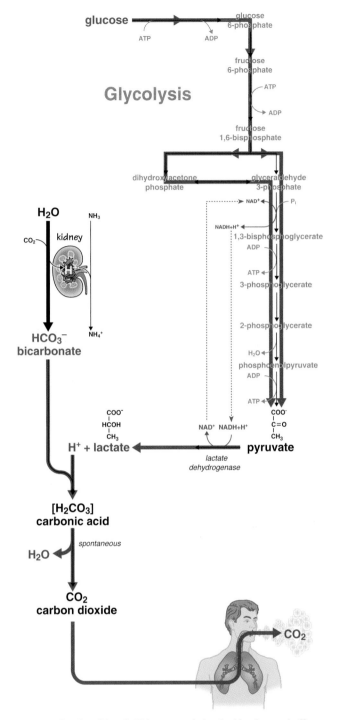

Figure 2.2 Lactic acid and pH homeostasis by the bicarbonate buffer system. The bicarbonate buffer system removes protons [H⁺] generated during anaerobic glycolysis. The protons are disposed of as water while the CO_2 evolved is expired via the lungs.

3 Production and removal of protons into and from the blood

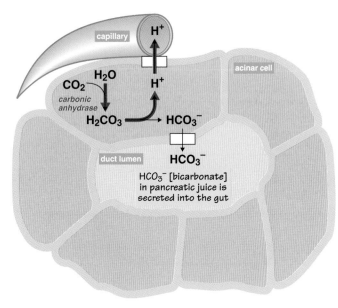

Figure 3.1 Secretion of protons into the blood by the acinar cell of the pancreas.

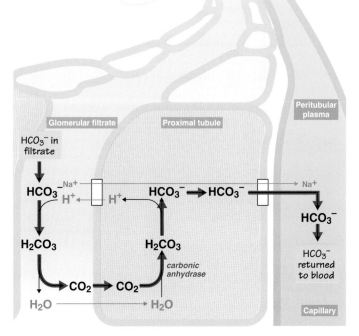

Figure 3.2 Reabsorption of bicarbonate from the renal glomerular filtrate into the blood.

The pancreas secretes protons into the blood
The acinar cells surrounding the pancreatic duct produce pancreatic juice. This contains a high concentration (up to 125 mmol/l) of HCO_3^- ions which when secreted into the gut neutralises the acidic products from the stomach. The secretion of HCO_3^- into the pancreatic juice is accompanied by an equivalent secretion of protons into the blood (Figure 3.1)

The role of the kidney in regulating blood proton concentration
The kidney plays a major role in regulating plasma pH. It (i) removes protons into the urine and (ii) regulates the concentration of plasma HCO_3^-
Bicarbonate reabsorption
Figure 3.2 shows how HCO_3^- is reabsorbed from the glomerular filtrate into the blood

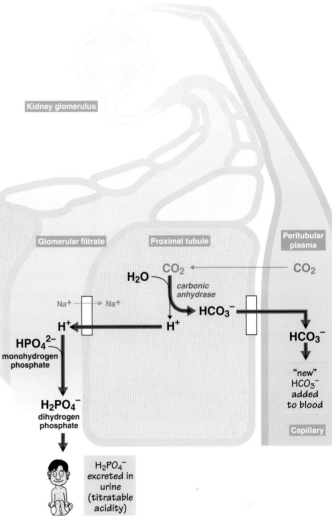

Figure 3.4 Production of "new" bicarbonate linked to excretion of dihydrogen phosphate ions.

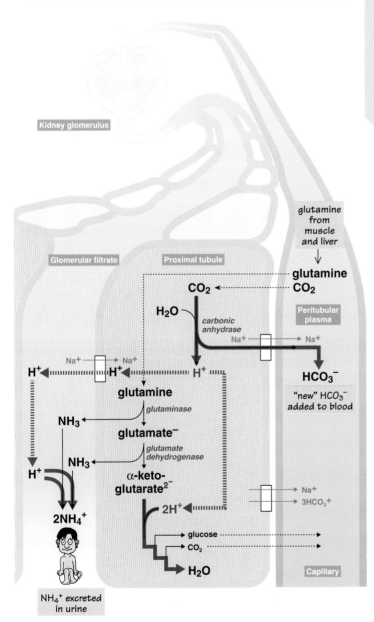

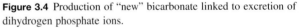

Figure 3.3 Production of "new" bicarbonate linked to excretion of ammonium ions.

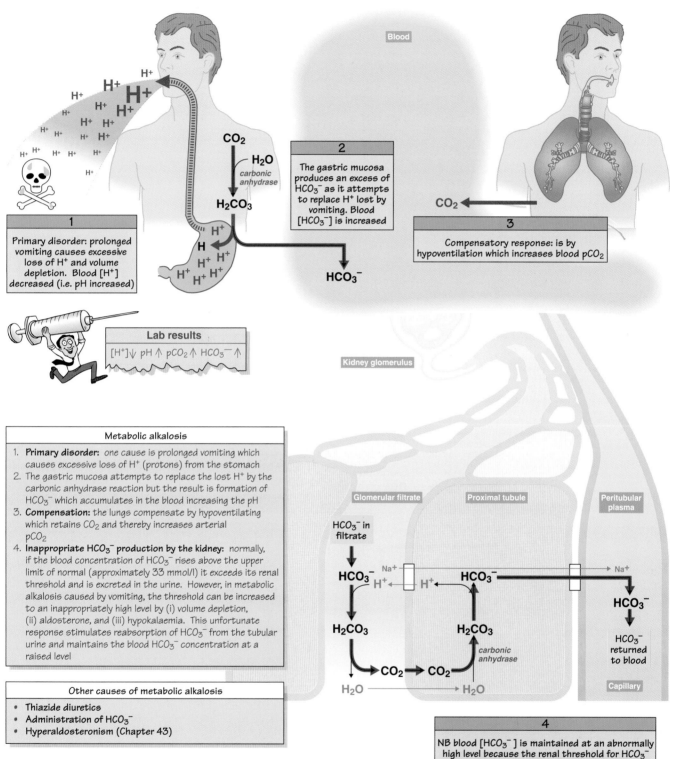

Blood

H^+ H^+ H^+ H^+ H^+ H^+ H^+ H^+ H^+ H^+ H^+ H^+ H^+ H^+ H^+ H^+

CO_2

H_2O
carbonic anhydrase

H_2CO_3

2
The gastric mucosa produces an excess of HCO_3^- as it attempts to replace H^+ lost by vomiting. Blood $[HCO_3^-]$ is increased

CO_2

1
Primary disorder: prolonged vomiting causes excessive loss of H^+ and volume depletion. Blood $[H^+]$ decreased (i.e. pH increased)

3
Compensatory response: is by hypoventilation which increases blood pCO_2

H^+ H H^+ H^+ H^+ H^+ H^+

HCO_3^-

Lab results
$[H^+]\downarrow$ pH $\uparrow$ $pCO_2\uparrow$ $HCO_3^-\uparrow$

Kidney glomerulus

Metabolic alkalosis

1. **Primary disorder:** one cause is prolonged vomiting which causes excessive loss of H^+ (protons) from the stomach
2. The gastric mucosa attempts to replace the lost H^+ by the carbonic anhydrase reaction but the result is formation of HCO_3^- which accumulates in the blood increasing the pH
3. **Compensation:** the lungs compensate by hypoventilating which retains CO_2 and thereby increases arterial pCO_2
4. **Inappropriate HCO_3^- production by the kidney:** normally, if the blood concentration of HCO_3^- rises above the upper limit of normal (approximately 33 mmol/l) it exceeds its renal threshold and is excreted in the urine. However, in metabolic alkalosis caused by vomiting, the threshold can be increased to an inappropriately high level by (i) volume depletion, (ii) aldosterone, and (iii) hypokalaemia. This unfortunate response stimulates reabsorption of HCO_3^- from the tubular urine and maintains the blood HCO_3^- concentration at a raised level

Other causes of metabolic alkalosis

- **Thiazide diuretics**
- **Administration of HCO_3^-**
- **Hyperaldosteronism (Chapter 43)**

Glomerular filtrate

Proximal tubule

Peritubular plasma

HCO_3^- in filtrate

HCO_3^-
H^+

Na^+

H^+

HCO_3^-

Na^+

H_2CO_3

H_2CO_3

HCO_3^-

CO_2 → CO_2

carbonic anhydrase

HCO_3^- returned to blood

H_2O → H_2O

Capillary

4
NB blood $[HCO_3^-]$ is maintained at an abnormally high level because the renal threshold for HCO_3^- (normally 23–33 mmol/l) is inappropriately increased in response to volume depletion

Figure 4.1 Metabolic alkalosis.

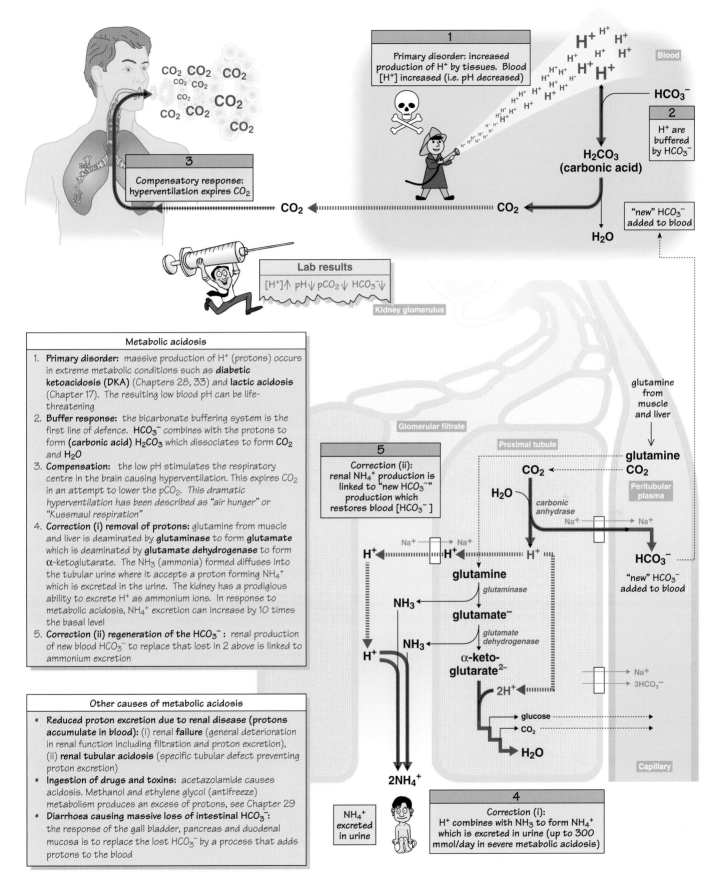

1

Primary disorder: increased production of H^+ by tissues. Blood $[H^+]$ increased (i.e. pH decreased)

2

H^+ are buffered by HCO_3^-

$H^+ + HCO_3^-$

H_2CO_3 (carbonic acid)

H_2O

"new" HCO_3^- added to blood

3

Compensatory response: hyperventilation expires CO_2

CO_2

Lab results

$[H^+]\uparrow\ pH\downarrow\ pCO_2\downarrow\ HCO_3^-\downarrow$

Kidney glomerulus

Blood

Metabolic acidosis

1. **Primary disorder:** massive production of H^+ (protons) occurs in extreme metabolic conditions such as **diabetic ketoacidosis (DKA)** (Chapters 28, 33) and **lactic acidosis** (Chapter 17). The resulting low blood pH can be life-threatening

2. **Buffer response:** the bicarbonate buffering system is the first line of defence. HCO_3^- combines with the protons to form **(carbonic acid)** H_2CO_3 which dissociates to form CO_2 and H_2O

3. **Compensation:** the low pH stimulates the respiratory centre in the brain causing hyperventilation. This expires CO_2 in an attempt to lower the pCO_2. *This dramatic hyperventilation has been described as "air hunger" or "Kussmaul respiration"*

4. **Correction (i) removal of protons:** glutamine from muscle and liver is deaminated by **glutaminase** to form **glutamate** which is deaminated by **glutamate dehydrogenase** to form α-ketoglutarate. The NH_3 (ammonia) formed diffuses into the tubular urine where it accepts a proton forming NH_4^+ which is excreted in the urine. The kidney has a prodigious ability to excrete H^+ as ammonium ions. In response to metabolic acidosis, NH_4^+ excretion can increase by 10 times the basal level

5. **Correction (ii) regeneration of the HCO_3^-:** renal production of new blood HCO_3^- to replace that lost in 2 above is linked to ammonium excretion

---

Other causes of metabolic acidosis

- **Reduced proton excretion due to renal disease (protons accumulate in blood):** (i) renal **failure** (general deterioration in renal function including filtration and proton excretion), (ii) **renal tubular acidosis** (specific tubular defect preventing proton excretion)

- **Ingestion of drugs and toxins:** acetazolamide causes acidosis. Methanol and ethylene glycol (antifreeze) metabolism produces an excess of protons, see Chapter 29

- **Diarrhoea causing massive loss of intestinal HCO_3^-:** the response of the gall bladder, pancreas and duodenal mucosa is to replace the lost HCO_3^- by a process that adds protons to the blood

---

5

Correction (ii): renal NH_4^+ production is linked to "new HCO_3^-" production which restores blood $[HCO_3^-]$

Glomerular filtrate

Proximal tubule

glutamine from muscle and liver

glutamine

CO_2

CO_2

H_2O

carbonic anhydrase

Peritubular plasma

$Na^+ \rightarrow Na^+$

$Na^+ \rightarrow Na^+$

$H^+ \rightarrow H^+$

H^+

HCO_3^-

"new" HCO_3^- added to blood

glutamine

NH_3

glutaminase

glutamate$^-$

NH_3

glutamate dehydrogenase

H^+

α-keto-glutarate^{2-}

$2H^+$

Na^+

$3HCO_3^-$

glucose

CO_2

H_2O

Capillary

$2NH_4^+$

NH_4^+ excreted in urine

4

Correction (i): H^+ combines with NH_3 to form NH_4^+ which is excreted in urine (up to 300 mmol/day in severe metabolic acidosis)

Figure 4.2 Metabolic acidosis.

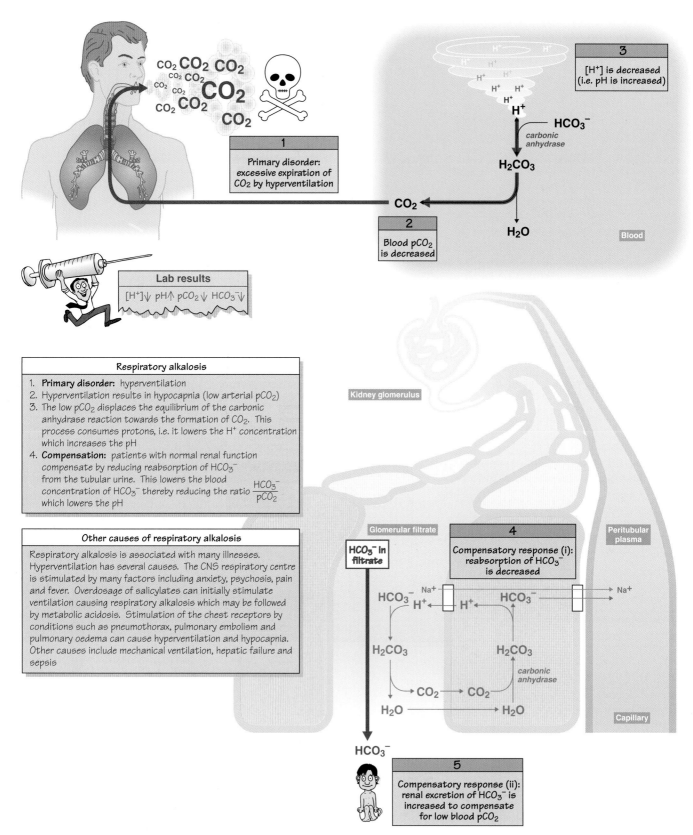

1

Primary disorder:
excessive expiration of
CO_2 by hyperventilation

2

Blood pCO_2
is decreased

3

$[H^+]$ is decreased
(i.e. pH is increased)

$$H^+ \longleftarrow HCO_3^-$$

carbonic anhydrase

$$H_2CO_3$$

$$CO_2 \quad H_2O$$

Blood

Lab results

$[H^+]\downarrow$ pH$\uparrow$ $pCO_2\downarrow$ $HCO_3^-\downarrow$

Respiratory alkalosis

1. **Primary disorder:** hyperventilation
2. Hyperventilation results in hypocapnia (low arterial pCO_2)
3. The low pCO_2 displaces the equilibrium of the carbonic anhydrase reaction towards the formation of CO_2. This process consumes protons, i.e. it lowers the H^+ concentration which increases the pH
4. **Compensation:** patients with normal renal function compensate by reducing reabsorption of HCO_3^- from the tubular urine. This lowers the blood concentration of HCO_3^- thereby reducing the ratio $\frac{HCO_3^-}{pCO_2}$ which lowers the pH

Other causes of respiratory alkalosis

Respiratory alkalosis is associated with many illnesses. Hyperventilation has several causes. The CNS respiratory centre is stimulated by many factors including anxiety, psychosis, pain and fever. Overdosage of salicylates can initially stimulate ventilation causing respiratory alkalosis which may be followed by metabolic acidosis. Stimulation of the chest receptors by conditions such as pneumothorax, pulmonary embolism and pulmonary oedema can cause hyperventilation and hypocapnia. Other causes include mechanical ventilation, hepatic failure and sepsis

Kidney glomerulus

Glomerular filtrate

HCO_3^- in
filtrate

Peritubular
plasma

4

Compensatory response (i):
reabsorption of HCO_3^-
is decreased

$$HCO_3^- \quad \overset{Na^+}{\underset{H^+}{}} \quad H^+ \quad HCO_3^- \quad \longrightarrow Na^+$$

$$H_2CO_3 \qquad\qquad H_2CO_3$$

carbonic anhydrase

$$CO_2 \longrightarrow CO_2$$

$$H_2O \longrightarrow H_2O$$

Capillary

HCO_3^-

5

Compensatory response (ii):
renal excretion of HCO_3^- is
increased to compensate
for low blood pCO_2

Figure 5.1 Respiratory alkalosis.

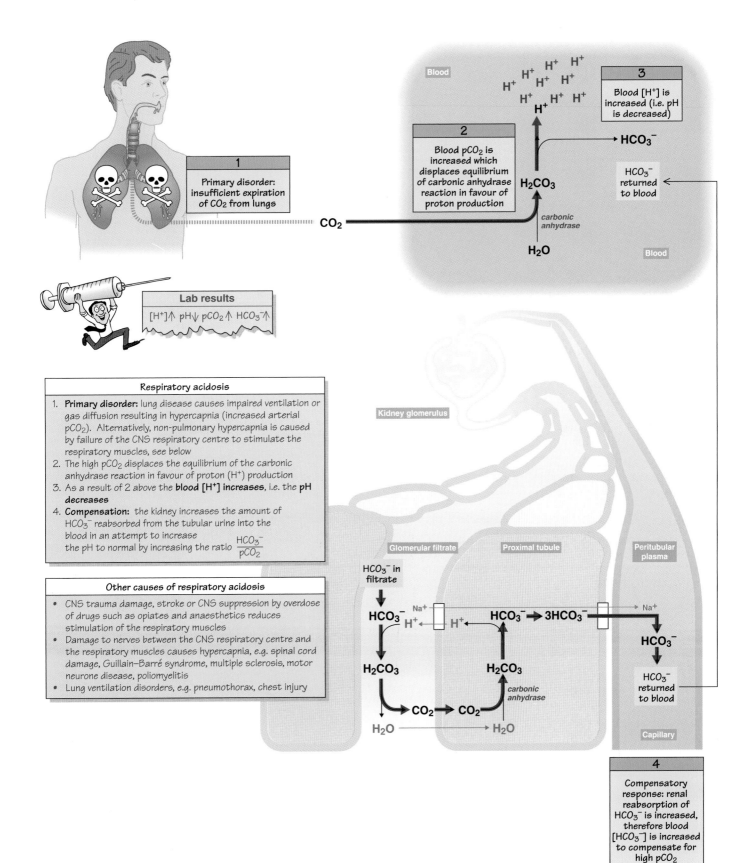

1
Primary disorder: insufficient expiration of CO₂ from lungs

2
Blood pCO₂ is increased which displaces equilibrium of carbonic anhydrase reaction in favour of proton production

3
Blood [H⁺] is increased (i.e. pH is decreased)

Blood

H_2CO_3

HCO_3^-

HCO_3^- returned to blood

carbonic anhydrase

H_2O

CO_2

Blood

Lab results

$[H^+]\uparrow$ $pH\downarrow$ $pCO_2\uparrow$ $HCO_3^-\uparrow$

Respiratory acidosis

1. **Primary disorder:** lung disease causes impaired ventilation or gas diffusion resulting in hypercapnia (increased arterial pCO_2). Alternatively, non-pulmonary hypercapnia is caused by failure of the CNS respiratory centre to stimulate the respiratory muscles, see below
2. The high pCO_2 displaces the equilibrium of the carbonic anhydrase reaction in favour of proton (H⁺) production
3. As a result of 2 above the **blood [H⁺] increases**, i.e. the **pH decreases**
4. **Compensation:** the kidney increases the amount of HCO_3^- reabsorbed from the tubular urine into the blood in an attempt to increase the pH to normal by increasing the ratio $\dfrac{HCO_3^-}{pCO_2}$

Other causes of respiratory acidosis

- CNS trauma damage, stroke or CNS suppression by overdose of drugs such as opiates and anaesthetics reduces stimulation of the respiratory muscles
- Damage to nerves between the CNS respiratory centre and the respiratory muscles causes hypercapnia, e.g. spinal cord damage, Guillain–Barré syndrome, multiple sclerosis, motor neurone disease, poliomyelitis
- Lung ventilation disorders, e.g. pneumothorax, chest injury

Kidney glomerulus

Glomerular filtrate   Proximal tubule   Peritubular plasma

HCO_3^- in filtrate

HCO_3^- Na⁺ $HCO_3^- \rightarrow 3HCO_3^-$ Na⁺
H⁺   H⁺

H_2CO_3 H_2CO_3 HCO_3^-

carbonic anhydrase

$CO_2 \rightarrow CO_2$

HCO_3^- returned to blood

$H_2O \rightarrow H_2O$

Capillary

4
Compensatory response: renal reabsorption of HCO_3^- is increased, therefore blood $[HCO_3^-]$ is increased to compensate for high pCO_2

Figure 5.2 Respiratory acidosis.

6 Amino acids and the primary structure of proteins

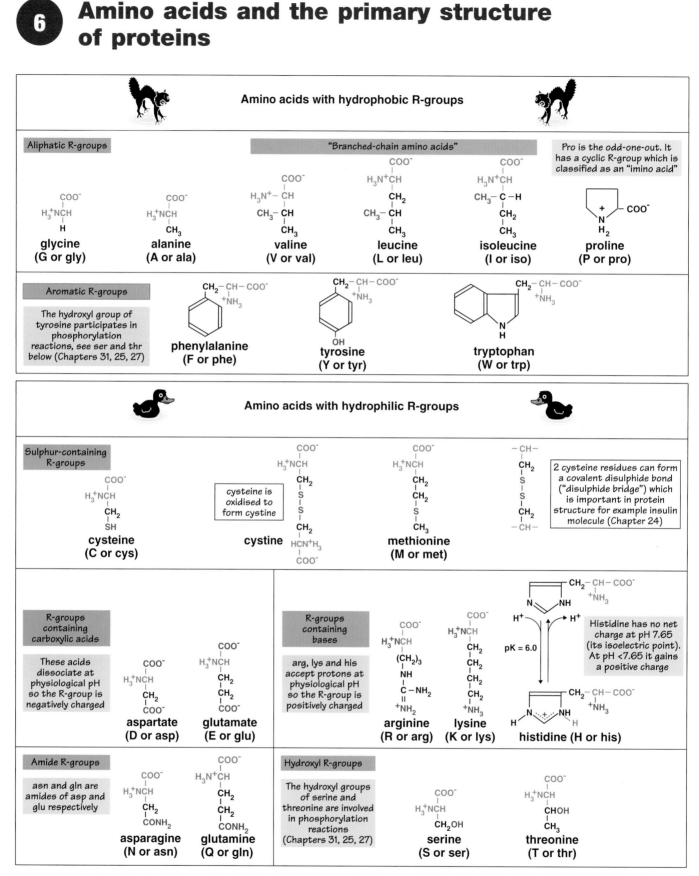

Figure 6.1 The amino acids classified according to their solubility in water. The R-group, which is either hydrophilic or hydrophobic, determines their solubility.

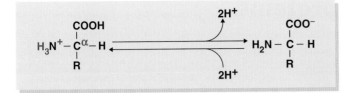

Figure 6.2 General structure of an amino acid.

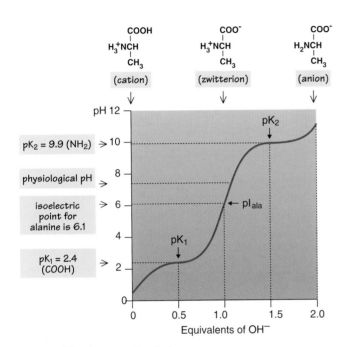

Figure 6.3 Titration curve for alanine.

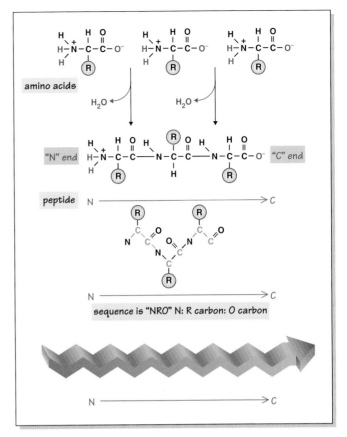

Figure 6.4 Primary structure of a protein. Polymerisation of amino acids to form a polypeptide chain. This is represented as a zig-zag with an arrow head at the C-terminus.

Amino acids

There are 20 amino acids that are the building blocks of proteins (Fig. 6.1). Amino acids are joined by peptide bonds in a precise order, which determines the **primary structure** of a protein.

Amino acids have an **α-carbon atom** with bonds to an **amino group**, a **carboxylic acid** group, a **hydrogen atom** and an "**R**" **group**, which is specific for each amino acid (Fig. 6.2). At physiological pH 7.4, the carboxylic acid dissociates to liberate a proton (**H⁺**) and form a carboxyl group (**COO⁻**), while the amino group accepts a proton (**H⁺**) to form (**NH₃⁺**). Thus at pH 7.4 an amino acid can have both a positive and a negative charge and is known as a **zwitterion** (from German, meaning hybrid ion). The dissociation of **alanine** is shown in its titration curve (Fig. 6.3).

At **low pH** (i.e. **high H⁺** concentration) the carboxyl and amino groups of alanine both **gain** an **H⁺**, giving the **cation** form (i.e. **neutral COOH** and positively charged **NH₃⁺**).

Mnemonic: a ca†ion has a†(positive) charge

At **high pH** (i.e. **low H⁺** concentration) the carboxyl and amino groups of alanine both **lose** an **H⁺**, giving the **anion** form (i.e. **negative COO⁻** and **neutral NH₂**).

Primary structure

Proteins are a specific sequence of amino acids arranged in a **polypeptide chain** that has an **N terminus** (**H₃N⁺**) and a **C terminus** (**COO⁻**) (Fig. 6.4). The amino acid sequence defines the **primary structure** and determines how the protein folds into its three-dimensional shape.

Secondary structure

Secondary structure largely depends on hydrogen bonding involving the peptide bonds, whereas tertiary structure (Chapter 8) depends on bonds involving the amino acid R-groups.

β-strands and β-sheets

The polypeptide chain is organised as **β-strands**. When several of these β-strands associate they form parallel or antiparallel **β-sheets** (Figs 7.1 and 7.2).

α-helices

Polypeptide chains associate by hydrogen bonds to form a **right-handed α-helix** (Fig. 7.3 *opposite*).

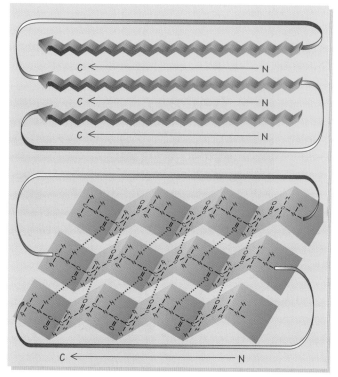

Figure 7.2 Parallel β-sheet. The three β-strands associate by hydrogen bonding to form a β-pleated sheet. The strands run in the same direction and so are described as being "parallel".

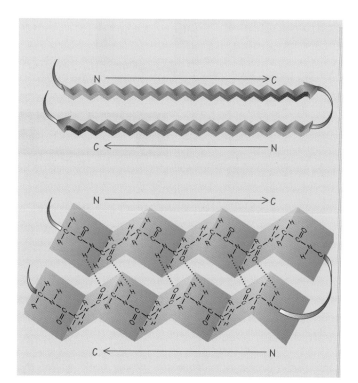

Figure 7.1 Antiparallel β-sheet. The polypeptide chains organise in a zig-zag manner to form β-strands. The β-strands can associate by hydrogen bonding to form a β-sheet. When two strands run in opposite directions, they are described as "antiparallel".

Abnormal primary structure affects the secondary structure: deletion of a single amino acid causes cystic fibrosis

The primary structure refers to the **amino acid sequence of the polypeptide chain**. An error caused by a single incorrect amino acid amongst a chain of 1480 amino acids can seriously affect the function of the protein. This happens in people with **cystic fibrosis** who have a defective **CFTR (cystic fibrosis transmembrane conductance regulator) gene**, which produces a defective chloride transporter protein. In 70% of people with cystic fibrosis, the mutation is deletion of 3 base pairs in the DNA, which results in the loss of phenylalanine

at position 508 (Fig. 7.4). This is known as the **ΔF508 mutation** (Δ for **deletion**; F for **phenylalanine**; 508 for the **position** of this phenylalanine in the primary structure). Following synthesis the abnormal CFTR protein folds into an incorrect **secondary structure** and is retained in the endoplasmic reticulum. Loss of the chloride transporter results in the accumulation of thick, viscous mucus, which adversely affects lung function. It also results in defective exocrine pancreatic secretion resulting in a malabsorption syndrome.

Altered secondary structure of a prion protein causes spongiform encephalopathy (e.g. CJD or "mad cow disease")

Prions are proteinaceous infectious particles consisting only of protein and do not contain DNA or RNA. Derangement of the secondary structure of prions results in the spongiform encephalopathies such a **scrapie** (in sheep) and **bovine spongiform encephalopathy (BSE or "mad cow disease")**. Human diseases are **Creutzfeldt–Jakob disease (CJD)**, **kuru** (from cannibalistic practice of eating human brain) and "**variant CJD**". Prion protein (PrP^C) is a normal cellular protein of unknown function that is expressed in neurones. As shown in Fig. 7.5, a prion normally consists mainly of **α-helices**. However, the **PrP^C** protein can be corrupted to the malignant form **PrP^{SC}** (^{SC} for **scrapie**), which comprises **mainly β-pleated sheets**. This in turn adversely affects the tertiary structure (see below) causing spongiform encephalopathy. The mechanism of the α-helix metamorphosis to a β-pleated sheet is not understood. The presence of an abnormal **PrP^SC** molecule somehow converts **PrP^C** molecules to **PrP^SC** molecules in a chain reaction which, like a rotten apple in a barrel, propagates disease throughout the brain.

Amyloidosis

Amyloidosis is a group of diseases in which **amyloid protein** accumulates. Amyloid was originally, but incorrectly, thought to be starch. In fact, it comprises proteins that have folded into **β-pleated sheets** forming extracellular deposits and, under polarised light, displaying **a characteristic apple-green birefringence of Congo red stain**. Twenty-three human proteins can form amyloid deposits. They are classified by the letter A (for **A**myloid) followed by the protein: e.g. **AL** (L for **L**ight chain of immunoglobins); A**β** (β-amyloid accumulates in **Alzheimer's disease**); A**TTR** (**TTR**: **T**rans**T**hy**R**etin protein which transports thyroxine and retinol); and A-**CAL** (CAL for **CAL**citonin).

Normal CFTR:

DNA bases —	ATC —	ATC —	TTT —	GGT —	GTT —
Amino acid	Ile	Ile	Phe	Gly	Val
Position	506	507	508	509	510

deleted in ΔF508 cystic fibrosis mutation

Cystic fibrosis ΔF508 CFTR:

DNA bases —	ATC —	ATT —	GGT —	GTT —
Amino acid	Ile	Ile	Gly	Val
Position	506	507	508	509

Figure 7.4 The ΔF508 mutation causes cystic fibrosis. Deletion of bases **CTT**, as shown, results in the loss of **phenylalanine** at position 508 from the **CFTR protein**, forming the dysfunctional product that causes cystic fibrosis. NB Isoleucine at 507 is not affected as both **ATC** and **ATT** code for isoleucine.

3.6 amino acids per turn of α-helix

Right-handed helix
Right hand with thumb pointing in direction of helix, fingers curled anticlockwise indicates a **right-handed helix**

Figure 7.3 Right-handed α-helix.

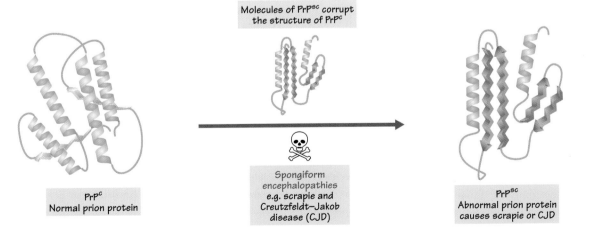

Molecules of PrP^sc corrupt the structure of PrP^c

PrP^c
Normal prion protein

Spongiform encephalopathies e.g. scrapie and Creutzfeldt–Jakob disease (CJD)

PrP^sc
Abnormal prion protein causes scrapie or CJD

Figure 7.5 Prion proteins. Normal prion protein (PrP^C) contains a lot of α-helical regions and is soluble. However, in the mutant prion that causes scrapie (PrP^SC), some of the α-helix is converted to the β-pleated conformation, which is insoluble. The mutant PrP^SC is "infectious" because it potentiates the conversion of an α-helix to β-conformation.

8 Tertiary and quaternary structure and collagen

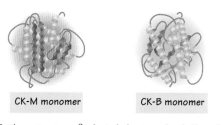

CK-M monomer   CK-B monomer

Figure 8.1 Tertiary structure. β-pleated sheets and α-helices fold themselves to form two different **creatine kinase (CK)** monomers (**CK-M** and **CK-B**).

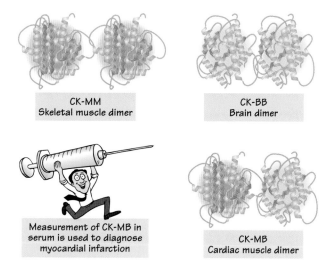

CK-MM
Skeletal muscle dimer

CK-BB
Brain dimer

Measurement of CK-MB in serum is used to diagnose myocardial infarction

CK-MB
Cardiac muscle dimer

Figure 8.2 Quaternary structure. The two different **creatine kinase** (CK) monomers (**M** and **B**) associate to form three different dimers: the **homo**-dimers **CK-MM** (found in skeletal muscle) and **CK-BB** (brain), and the **hetero**-dimer **CK-MB** (which is abundant in cardiac muscle).

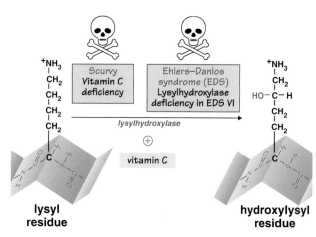

lysyl residue   hydroxylysyl residue

Figure 8.3 Hydroxylation of lysyl residue during collagen formation.

Tertiary structure of protein

When **β-strands**, **β-pleated sheets** and **α-helices** fold together they form the **tertiary** structure of the protein, for example the creatine kinase monomers CK-M and CK-B (Fig. 8.1).

Quaternary structure of protein

Many proteins consist of more than one polypeptide chain, which combine by non-covalent forces. The single protein is a **monomer**. The quaternary structure defines the association of monomers to form **dimers** (two monomers) (Fig. 8.2), **trimers** (three monomers), **tetramers** (four monomers), etc. and **oligomers** (composed of many monomers).

Collagen

Currently 19 types of collagen are known (Greek *kola*, glue); produces glue on boiling connective tissue. They are fibrous, structural proteins and are the most abundant protein in humans. Collagens are variably distributed, with type I being mainly found in ligaments, tendons and skin, and type II being the principal collagen in cartilage.

Collagen is constructed from **α-chain units** that associate to form a **triple helix**. The primary structure of collagen is repeats of the sequence **–Gly–X–Y–** where **X** is often proline. **Y** is usually a proline residue that has been hydroxylated in a vitamin C-dependent reaction producing a **hydroxyproline** residue. Alternatively, Y can be a **hydroxylysine** residue (Fig. 8.3). **Glycine** (remember its R-group is a single hydrogen atom) is an essential component because restricted space in the triple helix does not permit larger molecules.

Biosynthesis of collagen

Collagen is an extracellular, insoluble glycoprotein. This raises the question: how do **fibroblasts**, the collagen-producing cells, make an insoluble extracellular protein? The answer involves an intracellular stage and an extracellular stage (Fig. 8.4).

The intracellular stage produces procollagen

The intracellular protein-making machinery first of all produces polypeptide α-chains (approximately 1000 amino acids). Some of the prolyl and lysyl residues are hydroxylated by reactions that need vitamin C (Chapter 56). Some of the hydroxylysyl residues are glycosylated. The units then associate to form the triple helix (rope-like) **procollagen**, which is soluble.

The extracellular stage produces collagen fibres

Procollagen is secreted from the cell into the extracellular fluid where the terminal globular **propetides** are removed by **procollagen peptidase**, forming **tropocollagen**, which is insoluble. The tropocollagen units assemble into microfibrils in which each collagen unit is staggered so it overlaps its neighbours by one-quarter of the length of a collagen molecule. Finally, **lysyl oxidase** causes lysyl and hydroxylysyl residues to react, forming cross-links that provide tensile strength, and the microfibrils associate to form a polymeric collagen fibre.

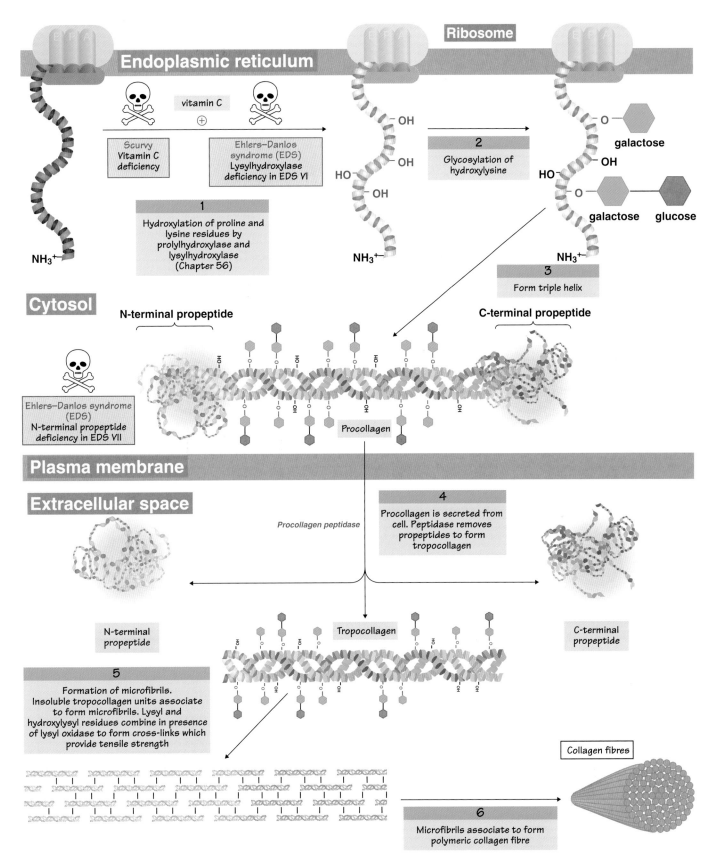

Endoplasmic reticulum

vitamin C
⊕

Scurvy
Vitamin C
deficiency

Ehlers–Danlos
syndrome (EDS)
Lysylhydroxylase
deficiency in EDS VI

1

Hydroxylation of proline and
lysine residues by
prolylhydroxylase and
lysylhydroxylase
(Chapter 56)

NH_3^+

— OH

— OH

HO —

— OH

NH_3^+

2

Glycosylation of
hydroxylysine

— O

galactose

— OH

HO —

— O

galactose   glucose

NH_3^+

3

Form triple helix

Cytosol

N-terminal propeptide

C-terminal propeptide

Ehlers–Danlos syndrome
(EDS)
N-terminal propeptide
deficiency in EDS VII

Procollagen

Plasma membrane

Extracellular space

Procollagen peptidase

4

Procollagen is secreted from
cell. Peptidase removes
propeptides to form
tropocollagen

N-terminal
propeptide

Tropocollagen

C-terminal
propeptide

5

Formation of microfibrils.
Insoluble tropocollagen units associate
to form microfibrils. Lysyl and
hydroxylysyl residues combine in presence
of lysyl oxidase to form cross-links which
provide tensile strength

Collagen fibres

6

Microfibrils associate to form
polymeric collagen fibre

Figure 8.4 Biosynthesis of collagen.

Oxidation/reduction reactions, coenzymes and prosthetic groups

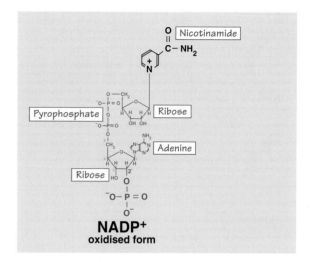

NAD⁺
oxidised form

NADH+H⁺
reduced form

Figure 9.1 NAD⁺ (nicotinamide adenine dinucleotide) is reduced to NADH.

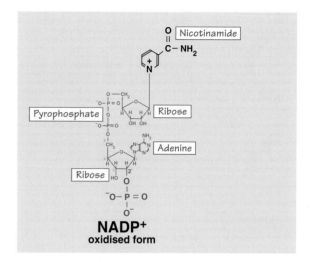

NADP⁺
oxidised form

Figure 9.2 NADP⁺ (nicotinamide adenine dinucleotide phosphate) is similar to NAD⁺ except for the ribose 2′-phosphate moiety. Similarly, NADP⁺ is reduced to NADPH (not shown).

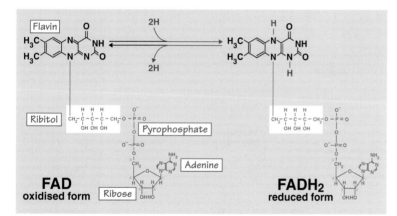

FAD
oxidised form

FADH₂
reduced form

Figure 9.3 FAD (flavin adenine dinucleotide) is reduced to FADH₂.

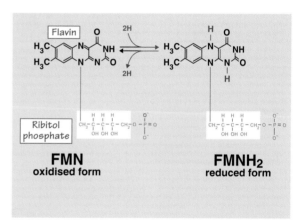

FMN
oxidised form

FMNH₂
reduced form

Figure 9.4 FMN (flavin mononucleotide) is reduced to FMNH₂.

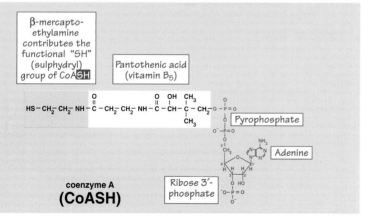

coenzyme A
(CoASH)

Figure 9.5 Coenzyme A. The SH (sulphydryl) group of β-mercaptoethylamine is the functional group that reacts, for example, with the carboxylate group of fatty acids.

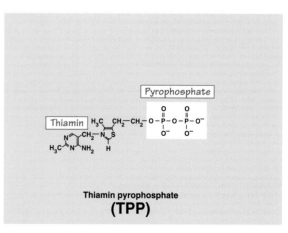

Thiamin pyrophosphate
(TPP)

Figure 9.6 Thiamin pyrophosphate.

The hydrogen carriers: coenzymes NAD$^+$ and NADP$^+$

NAD$^+$ and **NADP$^+$** (Figs 9.1 and 9.2) are coenzymes derived from niacin (Chapter 53) that function as co-substrates. Their job is to collaborate with enzyme X and collect the hydrogen from an oxidation reaction. In the process they are reduced to **NADH** and **NADPH**, respectively. Then, they say goodbye to enzyme X and diffuse away to collaborate with enzyme Y and donate hydrogen in a reducing reaction (in the process they are restored to their oxidised state: **NAD$^+$** and **NADP$^+$**).

NAD$^+$ and NADP$^+$, although very similar, have very different functions. **NADH is very important in energy metabolism** (e.g. Chapters 16 and 33) and **catabolic pathways**. **NADPH is very important in anabolic pathways**, e.g. fatty acid synthesis (Chapter 21) and the "respiratory burst" (Chapter 14).

NB MAJOR CONCEPT: coenzymes such as NAD$^+$, NADP$^+$ and coenzyme A must be recycled (Fig. 9.7)! They are derived from vitamins, are present in tiny quantities and when reduced they must be reoxidised in another enzyme reaction. Think of NAD$^+$ and NADP$^+$ as bees buzzing around the cell collecting hydrogen and then delivering it to a hydrogen user.

The prosthetic groups: FAD and FMN

FAD (Fig. 9.3) and **FMN** (Fig. 9.4) are enzyme co-factors derived from riboflavin (Chapter 53) and like NAD$^+$ and NADP$^+$ they collaborate as co-substrates in oxidation/reduction reactions and are reduced to **FADH$_2$** and **FMNH$_2$**. However, a major difference is that FAD and FMN are *not* coenzymes. They are **prosthetic groups**, meaning they are permanently attached to their enzymes by a covalent bond and therefore are a part of the enzyme structure.

Other coenzymes: coenzyme A and thiamin pyrophosphate

Coenzyme A and thiamin pyrophosphate are illustrated in Figs 9.5 and 9.6. For further details of other coenzymes see the chapters on vitamins (Chapters 53–56).

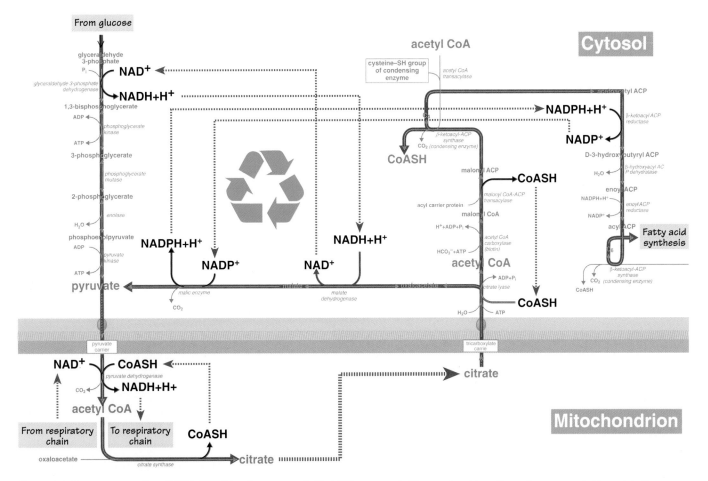

Figure 9.7 Coenzyme recycling. NAD$^+$, NADP$^+$ and coenzyme A (CoASH) are recycled in a partnership with another enzyme in the metabolic pathway. The pathway illustrated shows examples of coenzyme recycling when glucose is metabolised to fatty acids.

10 Anaerobic production of ATP by substrate-level phosphorylation, from phosphocreatine and by the adenylate kinase (myokinase) reaction

Adenosine triphosphate: the molecule that provides energy for living cells

The adenosine triphosphate (ATP) molecule is essential for life. It provides energy for muscle contraction, nerve conduction, many biochemical reactions, etc. At rest ATP turnover is 28 g (1 oz) of ATP per minute which is equivalent to 1.4 kg (3 lb) per hour. During strenuous exercise, ATP turnover increases to a massive 0.5 kg/min! Figure 10.1 shows that ATP consists of adenine, ribose and three phosphate groups that are identified as α-, β- and γ-. Hydrolysis of the "high energy" **phosphoanhydride bonds** between the **β- and γ-phosphorus** atoms, or alternatively, between the **α- and β-phosphorus** atoms releases energy for the biochemical reactions of life.

Quantitatively, the most efficient method for producing ATP is by **aerobic** metabolism by oxidative phosphorylation (Chapters 16 and 33). However, ATP can also be produced albeit less efficiently under **anaerobic** conditions by **substrate-level phosphorylation**, from **phosphocreatine**, and by the **adenylate kinase reaction**. Although less efficient, the ability to produce ATP without oxygen can be of life-saving importance.

Production of ATP by substrate-level phosphorylation

Figure 10.2 shows that ATP is formed by the **phosphoglycerate kinase** and **pyruvate kinase** glycolytic reactions; and in the Krebs cycle by **succinyl coenzyme A (CoA) synthetase** in co-operation with **nucleoside diphosphate kinase** (Fig. 10.3). *NB These reactions do not require oxygen.*

Production of ATP from phosphocreatine

Phosphocreatine is an important emergency reserve of "high energy" phosphate which rapidly produces ATP for muscle contraction anaerobically. This can be of life-saving significance but, unfortunately, this supercharge mechanism for ATP production lasts only for a few seconds.

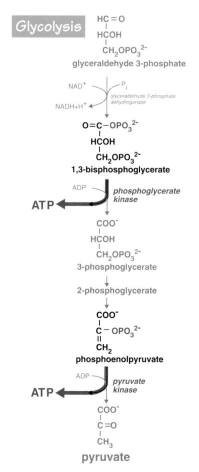

Figure 10.2 Substrate-level phosphorylation in glycolysis produces ATP.

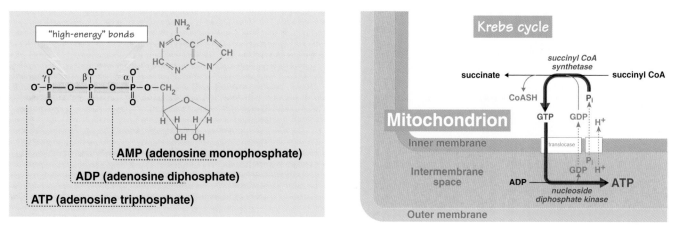

Figure 10.1 Structure of adenosine triphosphate (ATP).

Figure 10.3 Substrate-level phosphorylation in the Krebs cycle produces guanosine triphosphate (GTP), which is converted to ATP.

 Medical Biochemistry at a Glance, Third Edition. J. G. Salway. © 2012 John Wiley & Sons, Ltd. Published 2012 by John Wiley & Sons, Ltd.

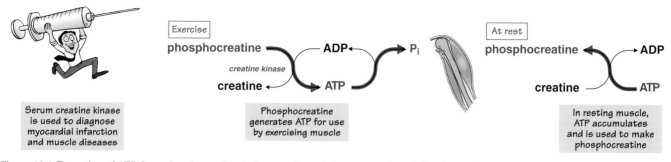

Figure 10.4 Formation of ATP from phosphocreatine during exercise and the regeneration of phosphocreatine from creatine during recovery.

During periods of rest when ATP is abundant, **creatine** is phosphorylated by **creatine kinase** to form phosphocreatine. This reaction is especially important in muscles. When a sudden explosive burst of muscle activity occurs, phosphocreatine phosphorylates adenosine diphosphate (ADP) to generate the ATP needed for muscle contraction (Fig. 10.4). For this reason, phosphocreatine is known as a "**phosphagen**".

Creatine is excreted as creatinine

Creatine is an amino acid but is not a component of proteins. It is made from arginine and is metabolised to **creatinine** prior to excretion in the urine (Chapter 44). Blood levels of creatinine and the creatinine clearance test are used to evaluate glomerular filtration in renal disease.

NB Do not be confused between **creatine**, **creatinine** *and* **carnitine**.

Creatine as an ergogenic aid

Ergogenic aids are substances that enhance the speed, power or stamina of an athlete, many of which are dangerous and illegal. Although controversial, a substantial body of opinion advocates **crea-**

$$ADP + ADP \xrightarrow[\text{(myokinase)}]{\text{adenylate kinase}} ATP + AMP$$

Figure 10.5 Formation of ATP from two molecules of ADP by the adenylate kinase reaction.

tine as the only ergogenic aid scientifically proven to enhance performance in both sprint and endurance events.

Production of ATP from ADP by adenylate kinase (myokinase)

When ATP has been hydrolysed to provide energy for muscle contraction, ADP accumulates. Remember that ADP still has a source of untapped energy in the α-phosphoanhydride bond (Fig. 10.1). With ingenious biochemical resourcefulness, this energy is salvaged when two molecules of ADP form ATP under anaerobic conditions using the **adenylate kinase** reaction (previously known as myokinase) (Fig. 10.5).

11 Aerobic production of ATP

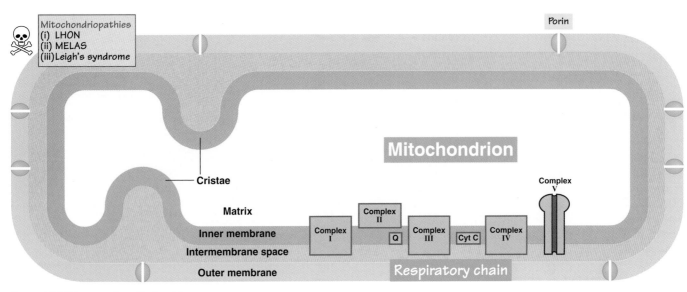

Figure 11.1 Diagram of a mitochondrion.

Production of ATP by oxidative phosphorylation in the respiratory chain
Mitochondrion

The mitochondrion (Fig. 11.1) is an organelle approximately the size of a bacterium. It is notable for having two membranes: an **outer membrane** that contains **porin** molecules rendering it permeable to molecules smaller than 10 kDa and an **inner membrane** that is **EXTREMELY IMPERMEABLE** and is folded into cristae. Although small molecules such as H_2O and NH_3 can cross the inner membrane, carrier proteins and shuttle systems enable a few exclusive molecules to cross this barrier.

It is postulated that the inner membrane and its contents are derived from an ancient aerobic bacterium that invaded a primitive cell during the early stages of evolution and is an example of endosymbiosis. A relic from the past is that the mitochondrion has its own DNA (mtDNA) encoding 37 genes. Of these, 24 are needed for mtDNA translation and the rest encode proteins of the respiratory chain. Notably only 13 of the more than 85 proteins composing the mitochondrial respiratory chain are encoded in mtDNA. The others are encoded by the nuclear DNA and imported from the cytoplasm.

Respiratory chain

The respiratory chain (Fig. 11.2 *opposite*) is a very efficient pathway for producing ATP from NADH and $FADH_2$, which in turn are formed by the oxidation of metabolic fuels, especially carbohydrates and fatty acids (Chapters 16 and 33). The respiratory chain consists of: complex I, complex II, complex III, complex IV and a mushroom-shaped multicomplex (complex V) comprising F_1 (fraction "one") and F_O (fraction "oh") that binds oligomycin. Some of these complexes contain cytochromes that transport electrons along the chain. Complex III contains cytochrome b, while complex IV contains cytochrome a/a_3. Ubiquinone (Q, coenzyme Q10) and cytochrome c (Cyt c) also participate in electron transfer. The complexes are located in the mitochondrial inner membrane. Complexes I, III and IV not only transfer electrons but also pump protons into the intermembrane space. The inner membrane is very impermeable and, in particular, it is impermeable to protons. The protons can return to the matrix only by passing through the F_1/F_O complex, which generates ATP.

The flow of electrons is shown simplistically in Fig. 11.2. Chapter 12 illustrates how the flow of electrons (electric current) powers the proton pumps. Finally, the respiratory chain is shown in cartoon form in Fig. 13.1.

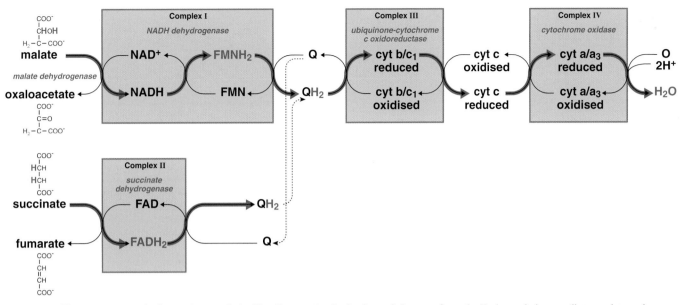

Figure 11.2 Electron transport in the respiratory chain. The diagram details the flow of electrons from the Krebs cycle intermediates malate and succinate via the electron transport chain (complexes I, II, III and IV) to oxygen.

Mitochondriopathies

There are several disorders of the respiratory chain. Many are transmitted by maternal inheritance as generally all mitochondria in the ovum are of maternal origin. The thousands of mtDNA molecules in one cell are distributed randomly to the daughter cells, therefore different tissues may harbour a mixture of both normal and mutant mtDNA (heteroplasmy). Accordingly the clinical phenotype is highly variable. Mutations in nuclear genes encoding proteins for the respiratory chain are transmitted autosomally and usually cause a more severe disease.

Leber hereditary optic neuropathy (LHON)

LHON is caused by a **mutation in the mitochondrial DNA** encoding one of the **complex I** subunits. It appears that the optic nerve is especially vulnerable to this respiratory chain dysfunction. This condition occurs in adults and results in loss of vision.

Mitochondrial encephalopathy, lactic acidosis and stroke-like episodes (MELAS)

MELAS is caused by a **mitochondrial DNA mutation** of the gene encoding leucine transfer RNA. This mutation affects translation of mitochondrial DNA so **all the respiratory chain complexes** are impaired with the exception of complex II, which is totally encoded in the nucleus.

Leigh's syndrome

Leigh's syndrome is an early-onset, degenerative, neurological disorder with characteristic neuropathological changes. Genetically, it is **heterogeneous** and is caused mainly by abnormal components of the respiratory chain encoded by **nuclear genes**; however, **mitochondrial gene** abnormalities also occur. The activity of **ATP synthetase (complex V) or complexes I, II, III and IV can be impaired**. There are also forms of Leigh's syndrome that have **abnormal pyruvate dehydrogenase (PDH)** complex activity (Chapter 32).

PDH deficiency results in raised blood concentrations of pyruvate, lactate and alanine. Some patients respond to supplementation with lipoic acid or thiamin (coenzymes for PDH). Treatment with a low carbohydrate, ketogenic diet has been advocated but with limited success. *(The ketone bodies readily cross the blood–brain barrier and their catabolism produces acetyl CoA independently of PDH.)*

12 Biosynthesis of ATP by oxidative phosphorylation I

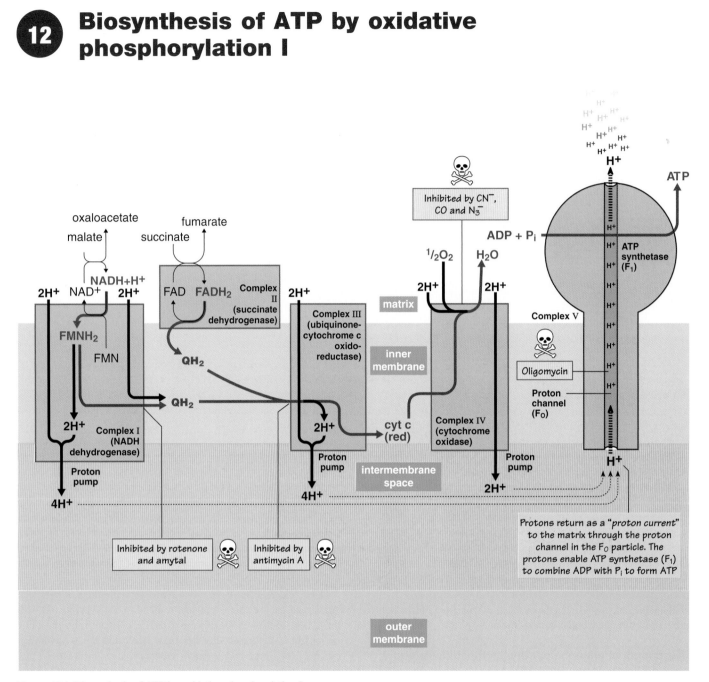

Figure 12.1 Biosynthesis of ATP by oxidative phosphorylation I.

The biosynthesis of ATP involves the flow of both electrons (e^-) and protons (H^+) in the respiratory chain to form ATP by the process known as **oxidative phosphorylation**. The respiratory chain comprises four structures known as **complex I**, **complex II**, **complex III** and **complex IV**; and a mushroom-shaped structure (**ATP synthetase** alias F_O/F_1 or **complex V**) that synthesises ATP from ADP and inorganic phosphate (Pi). We will consider the flow of electrons and protons: (i) first from complex I, and (ii) from complex II.

Complex I
Starting from NADH+H⁺: The energy for ATP synthesis is provided when charge separation in complex I generates a current of **electrons** (electricity) and a current of **protons** ("protonicity"). Four protons are

pumped into the intermembrane space. These protons, together with those pumped by complexes III and IV, form an electrochemical gradient, eventually flowing back through the proton channel of ATP synthetase (see below). The electrons (and two protons) reduce ubiquinone (coenzyme **Q**) to ubiquinol (**QH₂**), which diffuses through the membrane to **complex III**.

Complex II
Starting from FADH₂: Complex II contains FAD as the prosthetic group of several dehydrogenases, e.g. succinate dehydrogenase, and is reduced to FADH₂. Complex II conducts electrons to Q for onward transport to complex III. NB Complex II does not pump protons.

Complex III

Electrons are received from QH_2, which is oxidised back to Q, which is now able to return to transport another pair of electrons and protons. The electrons are passed to **cytochrome c** which transports them to complex IV. Complex III extrudes four protons by its proton pump.

Complex IV

Electrons received from cytochrome c are conducted to oxygen, which is reduced to form water. Complex IV extrudes only two protons.

ATP synthetase (complex V)

This complex consists of the "stem of the mushroom" F_O (**f**raction sensitive to **o**ligomycin) that contains the proton channel, and the "bulbous part" ATP synthetase (or F_1, the **1**st **f**raction to be discovered). The proton current flows through the **proton channel** and drives a molecular motor that causes ADP and Pi to react to form ATP.

Since a total of **four protons is needed to form one molecule of ATP** and transport it to the cytosol, **NADH+H^+** when oxidised can **extrude ten protons**, which can **generate 2.5 molecules of ATP**. Similarly, oxidation of **$FADH_2$** results in the **extrusion** of **six protons** that can **generate 1.5 molecules of ATP**.

Leakage of electrons produces reactive oxygen species

Approximately 2% of the electrons escape from the respiratory chain and combine directly with oxygen to form reactive oxygen species (ROS) (Chapter 14). If respiratory chain function is impaired even more, ROS are formed. These ROS damage the mitochondria and a vicious circle ensues resulting in ageing.

Respiratory poisons

Compounds that inhibit ATP production are, not surprisingly, potent toxins.

Amytal and **rotenone** inhibit electron transport at **complex I**. Rotenone is a natural pesticide extracted from the derris plant and so is popular with "organic" gardeners, with some justification as it is poorly absorbed from the gastrointestinal tract in humans and is therefore relatively harmless. However, it is rapidly absorbed through the gills of fish and so is notoriously toxic to them. Chronic exposure to rotenone in humans reproduces Parkinson's disease.

Antimycin inhibits electron transport at **complex III**.

Cyanide (CN^-), carbon monoxide (CO) and **azide (N_3^-)** inhibit **complex IV**. Hence, in cases of cyanide poisoning, despite the blood of the subjects being well oxygenated, they are incapable of aerobic metabolism. Consequently, their venous blood is red and similar in colour to their arterial blood. Also, lactic acid accumulates and stimulates the respiratory centre, causing hyperventilation.

Oligomycin blocks the **proton channel (F_O of complex V)** preventing the return flow of protons to the matrix and therefore the production of ATP by **ATP synthetase (F_1)**.

Dinitrophenol uncouples oxidative phosphorylation (Chapter 14).

13 Biosynthesis of ATP by oxidative phosphorylation II

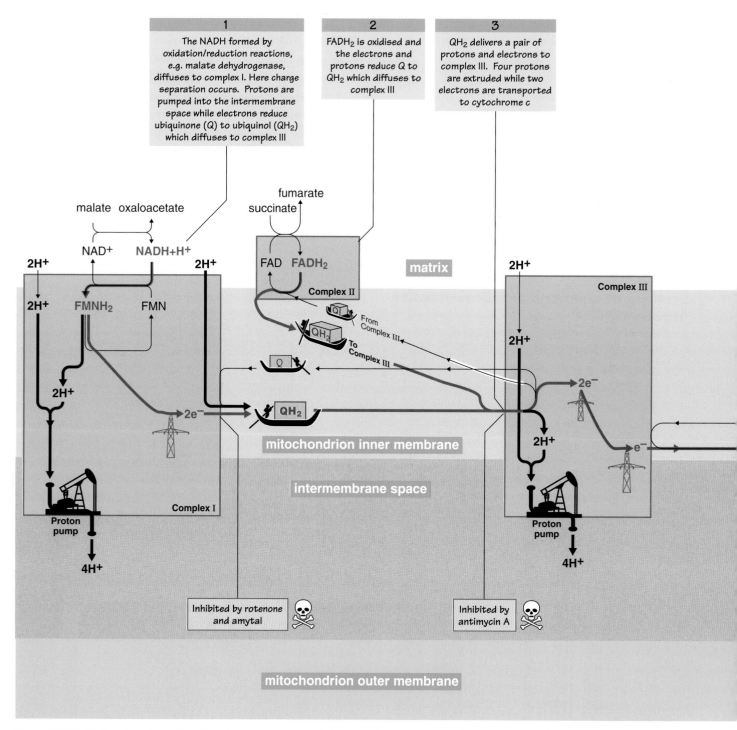

Figure 13.1 Oxidative phosphorylation. A cartoon representation of electron and proton transport via the respiratory chain which produces ATP by oxidative phosphorylation. A concise version of this diagram, which is more appropriate for examination purposes, is shown in Chapter 11, Fig. 11.2.

The flow of electrons and protons from **NADH+H⁺** and **FADH₂** via **complexes I and II**, respectively, to **complex III** of the respiratory chain are shown in Fig. 13.1. Electrons are then transported to **complex IV** where they combine with oxygen. Meanwhile, protons are pumped into the intermembrane space and are returned to the matrix via the proton channel in the F_O subunit of ATP synthetase (complex V). The flow of protons ("protonicity") drives a molecular motor in the **ATP synthetase** complex (F_1 particle) which aligns molecules of **ADP** and **Pi** so they combine to form **ATP**.

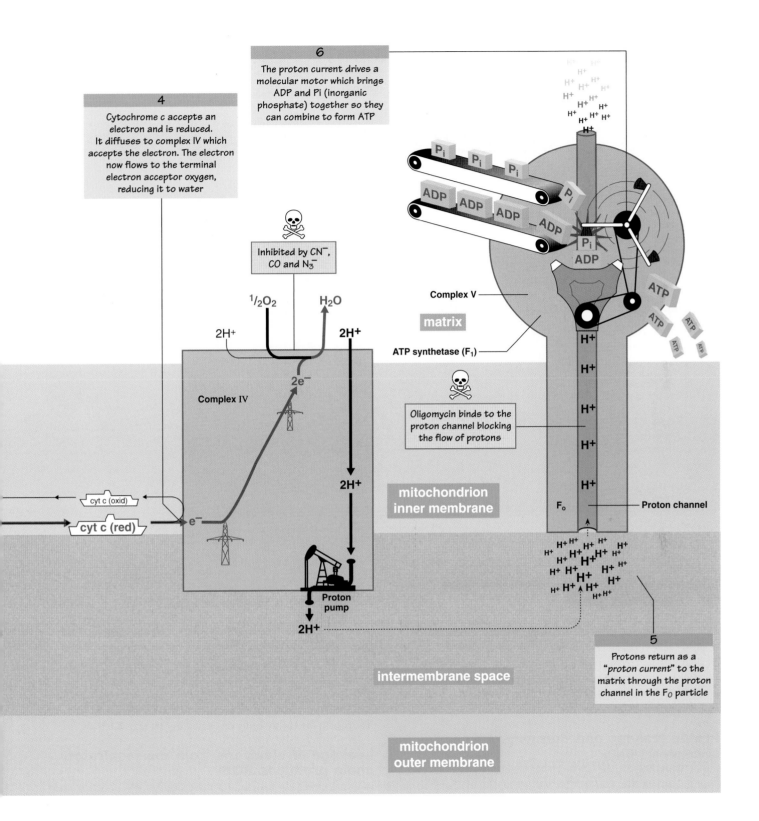

4

Cytochrome c accepts an electron and is reduced. It diffuses to complex IV which accepts the electron. The electron now flows to the terminal electron acceptor oxygen, reducing it to water

6

The proton current drives a molecular motor which brings ADP and Pi (inorganic phosphate) together so they can combine to form ATP

☠ Inhibited by CN^-, CO and N_3^-

$^1/_2O_2$ H_2O

$2H^+$ $2H^+$

$2e^-$

Complex IV

$2H^+$

☠ Oligomycin binds to the proton channel blocking the flow of protons

Complex V

matrix

ATP synthetase (F_1)

H^+
H^+
H^+
H^+
H^+

ADP   ADP   ADP   ADP

P_i P_i P_i P_i P_i

H^+

ADP

ATP   ATP   ATP   ATP   ATP

cyt c (oxid)

cyt c (red) e^-

F_o **Proton channel**

mitochondrion inner membrane

Proton pump

$2H^+$

H^+ H^+ H^+ H^+ H^+
H^+ H^+ H^+ H^+ H^+
H^+ H^+ H^+ H^+
H^+ H^+ H^+ H^+
H^+ H^+

5

Protons return as a "proton current" to the matrix through the proton channel in the F_O particle

intermembrane space

mitochondrion outer membrane

What happens when protons or electrons leak from the respiratory chain?

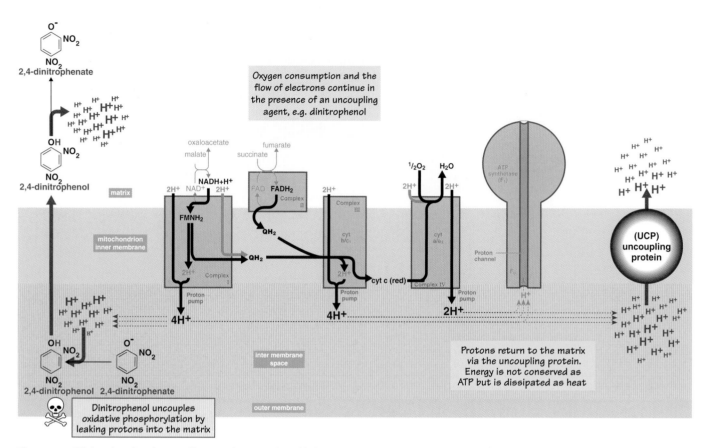

Figure 14.1 Dinitrophenol and uncoupling protein uncouple oxidative phosphorylation from electron transport.

Leakage of protons or electrons from the respiratory chain

We have seen in the previous pages how the formation of ATP from ADP by oxidative phosphorylation depends on both a flow of protons (a proton current) and a flow of electrons (an electron current). Inevitably there will be consequences if leakage of either protons or electrons occurs. **Proton leakage is associated with thermogenesis. Electron leakage is associated with the formation of reactive oxygen species (ROS)**, which can be extremely toxic.

Proton leakage and thermogenesis
Dinitrophenol (DNP)
During World War I, some workers in the ammunition factories developed fevers and lost weight. This was eventually attributed to the explosive they were handling called dinitrophenol (**DNP**). The ability of DNP to "speed up the metabolic rate" was exploited as a slimming pill until it was banned in the 1930s because of its adverse side effects. DNP causes protons to leak from the intermembrane space to the matrix thus bypassing the **ATP synthetase** system (Fig. 14.1).

DNP is an "uncoupling agent" and **uncouples electron transport from oxidative phosphorylation**. It does this when the **dinitrophenate anion** accepts a proton to form **dinitrophenol**, which is lipid soluble, and diffuses across the mitochondrial inner membrane. When

it reaches the matrix, it dissociates releasing its proton. The energy that otherwise would have been used for ATP synthesis is dissipated as heat (hence the fevers experienced by the ammunition workers).

Uncoupling protein
Uncoupling protein 1 (**UCP1**; originally called **thermogenin**) is found only in mammalian brown adipose tissue and is responsible for cold-induced, non-shivering thermogenesis. It performs this function by enabling protons to leak from the intermembrane space into the matrix with the energy being dissipated as heat (Fig. 14.1).

Leakage of electrons from the respiratory chain produces ROS

ROS are extremely toxic and a more detailed description of their production and devastating effects is provided in Chapter 15. (*Readers might prefer to study Chapter 15 before returning to this text.*)

The respiratory chain is the major source of ROS
In theory, molecular oxygen should be **completely reduced** in complex IV by four electrons to form water without the formation of intermediates. **In practice**, occasionally, **partial reduction** occurs with oxygen being converted to **superoxide anion radicals** (Chapter 15). Also, the ubiquinone reactions in complexes I and II have an

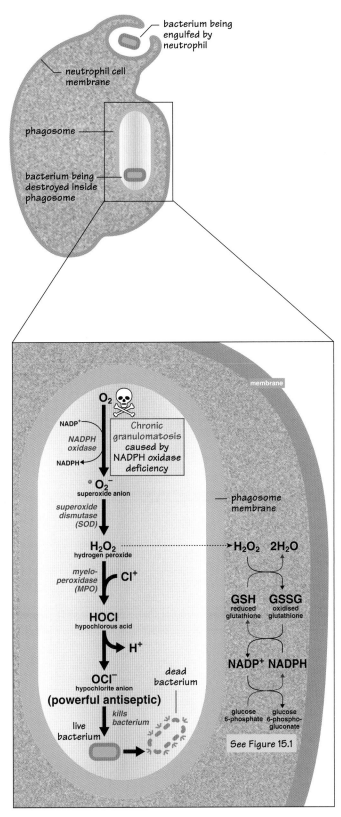

Figure 14.2 The respiratory burst in phagocytes kills bacteria.

unfortunate tendency to leak electrons directly to oxygen. Overall up to 2% of cellular oxygen forms superoxide free radicals and the body has developed defence mechanisms such as **superoxide dismutase**, **glutathione reductase** and **catalase** to dispose of them.

ROS as "good guys": the "respiratory burst" makes bleach!

Although ROS are extremely toxic, this can be used to the body's advantage, as exemplified by the "**respiratory burst**". The respiratory burst is a sudden surge of aerobic metabolism producing **hypochlorous acid** which is used to kill pathogens (Fig. 14.2).

Phagocytic cells such as macrophages and neutrophils defend the body against pathogens with microbiocidal peptides and lytic enzymes. They also produce microbiocidal oxidants whose formation is accompanied by a transient episode of oxidative metabolism known as the respiratory burst (see Figs 14.2 and 15.1 for more details). The neutrophil engulfs the pathogen in a membrane-enclosed **phagosome** and **NADPH oxidase** is activated on the phagosomal membrane, producing **superoxide anions**. These are converted to oxygen and hydrogen peroxide by **superoxide dismutase** (**SOD**). In neutrophils (but not macrophages), **myeloperoxidase** catalyses the oxidation of chloride ions by hydrogen peroxide, forming **hypochlorous acid** (yes, the swimming pool sanitiser and domestic bleach!), and this dissociates forming **hypochlorite ions**, which kill the pathogens.

Chronic granulomatous disease (**CGD**) is a rare, X-linked deficiency of NADPH oxidase activity that drastically impairs the ability of macrophages and neutrophils to destroy pathogens. Patients are especially vulnerable to infection by *Mycobacteria*, *Escherichia coli* and staphylococci since these organisms produce catalase to defend themselves against hydrogen peroxide attack by the phagocytes.

Free radicals, reactive oxygen species and oxidative damage

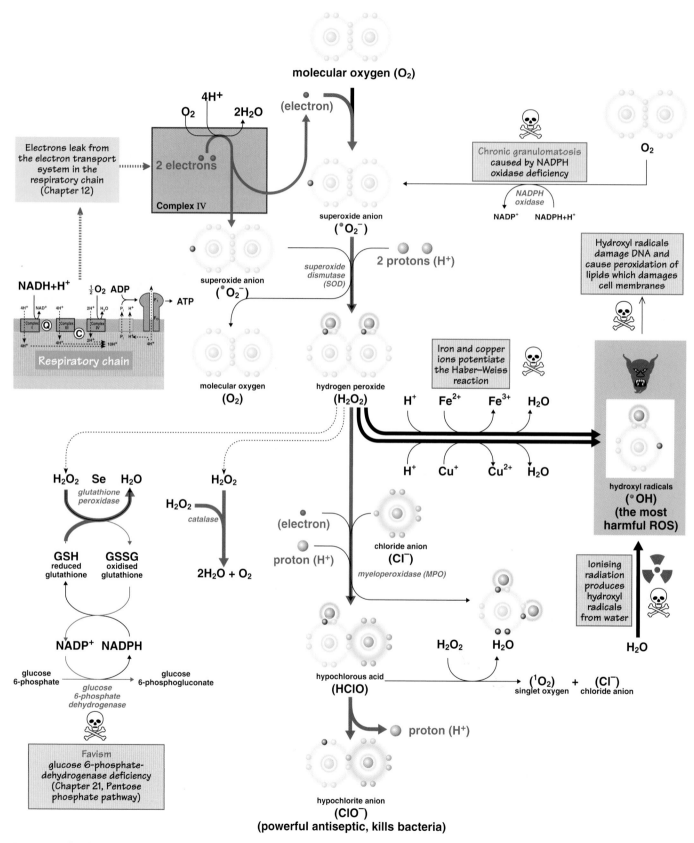

Figure 15.1 Production of free radicals and reactive oxygen species.

Reactive oxygen species and free radicals

Reactive oxygen species (ROS) is a term that describes: (i) **free radicals**, e.g. the hydroxyl radical $^\bullet OH$ (NB it differs from the hydroxyl ion OH^-); (ii) **ions**, e.g. the hypochlorite ion ClO^-, the conjugate base formed from the dissociation of hypochlorous acid and the active component of domestic bleach; (iii) a **combined free radical and ion**, e.g. the superoxide anion $^\bullet O_2^-$; or (iv) **molecules**, e.g. hydrogen peroxide H_2O_2.

A free radical is any species capable of independent existence with at least one unpaired electron (shown as $^\bullet$) in its outer orbit. Free radicals are very unstable, short-lived molecules that react rapidly with adjacent molecules causing cellular damage. Particularly prone are unsaturated fats leading to the process of lipid peroxidation, DNA damage and protein modification. They do this by stealing an electron from a neighbouring molecule to partner one of their own unpaired electrons. That would be fine except that the neighbouring molecule now has a lone electron and has become a free radical! A breakdown of molecular law and order results in a chain reaction of neighbour stealing an electron from its neighbour, and the result can be damage to the cell.

Production of free radicals
Respiratory chain

The respiratory chain is the major source of oxygen free radicals. **In theory**, molecular oxygen should be **completely reduced** in complex IV by four electrons from water without the formation of intermediates. **In practice**, sometimes **partial reduction** occurs with oxygen being converted to superoxide anion radicals (Fig. 15.1). Also, the ubiquinone reactions in complexes I and II have an unfortunate tendency to leak electrons directly to oxygen. Overall, up to 2% of cellular oxygen forms superoxide free radicals and the body has developed defence mechanisms to counter their damaging effects.

Ionising radiation

The interaction of ionising radiation with H_2O and O_2 generates free radicals. However, although they can be harmful to normal cells, during radiotherapy when they are focused on cancer cells in a high-dose target zone, lethal free-radical-mediated damage to the cancer cell DNA occurs.

Pollutants

Tobacco smoke contains epoxides and peroxides that may react with and damage the alveoli. The tar contains free radicals derived from quinones and semiquinones. Inhalation of inorganic particles such as asbestos causes free-radical-mediated lung damage.

Myocardial ischaemia and reperfusion-induced injury

Reperfusion to restore the flow of oxygenated blood to ischaemic tissue is essential for its survival but it produces oxygen free radicals, which are thought to be responsible for reperfusion-induced injury.

Metal ions

The transition metals, especially copper and iron ions, catalyse the formation of harmful hydroxyl radicals ($^\bullet OH$) from hydrogen peroxide (**Haber–Weiss reaction**). Because iron mediates oxidative damage, the substantial intracellular pool of free iron must be regulated by iron chelators, e.g. intracellular storage proteins such as ferritin.

Free radicals: friend or foe?
Free radicals as friends

Free radicals are not always the bad guys! **Nitric oxide ($NO^\bullet$)** is produced by the endothelial cells to control blood pressure, **hydrogen peroxide** is needed to make thyroxine, and phagocytes produce **ROS** that kill pathogens using the **respiratory burst** (Chapter 14).

Free radicals as foes

Free radicals usually are bad guys. They cause peroxidation damage to lipids, damage DNA causing cancer, and inflict oxidative damage on the body's tissues, contributing to premature ageing and many degenerative diseases especially cardiovascular disease. The most harmful are hydroxyl radicals ($^\bullet OH$).

Defence mechanisms against free radicals and reactive oxygen species
Enzymic defences

As shown in Fig. 15.1, **superoxide dismutase (SOD)** dismutes superoxide anions to hydrogen peroxide, which is safely converted to water and molecular oxygen by **catalase**. Furthermore, hydrogen peroxide is disposed of by cytosolic **glutathione peroxidase**, a **selenium-dependent** enzyme that provides a major route for elimination.

Free radical scavengers

Free radical scavengers are molecules that react with free radicals and render them harmless. There is considerable interest in foods rich in vitamins A, C and E (Chapters 51, 52 and 56) and those with an abundance of phytochemicals such as the phenols, polyphenols and flavonoids, which have high **oxygen radical absorbance capacity (ORAC)** values. These are potent free radical scavengers that are thought to reduce the risk of several chronic degenerative disorders.

Oxygen radical absorbance capacity values

Recently there has been popular interest in the beneficial effects of foods with high ORAC values. ORAC values are an assessment of the total antioxidant content of foods (including, for example, phenols and vitamins C and E) assessed as mmol TE/kg, where TE is "Trolox equivalent". Trolox® is a water-soluble analogue of vitamin E with potent antioxidant properties used as a reference compound for *in vitro* food tests.

Aerobic oxidation of glucose to provide energy as ATP

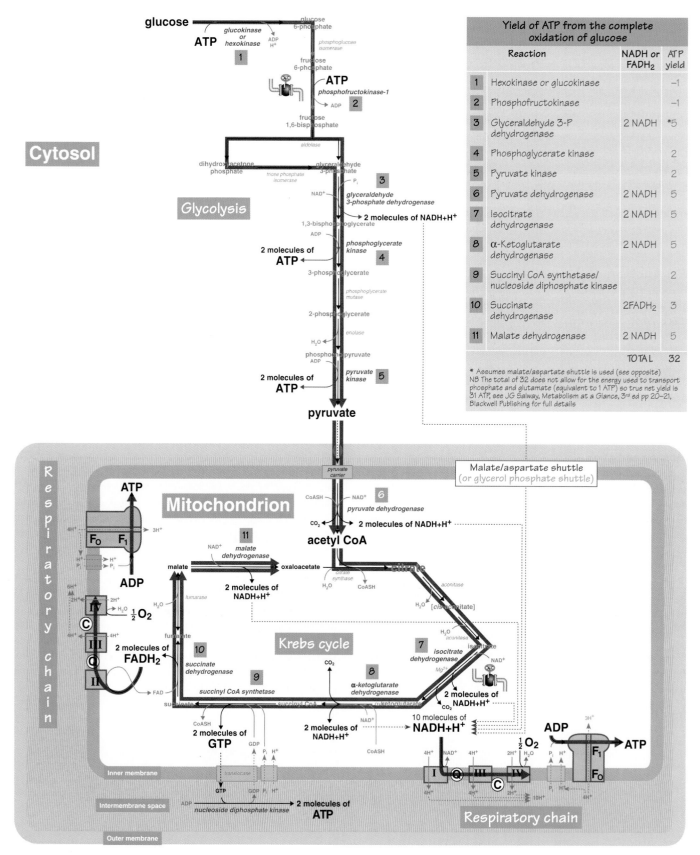

Yield of ATP from the complete oxidation of glucose		
Reaction	NADH or FADH$_2$	ATP yield
1 Hexokinase or glucokinase		–1
2 Phosphofructokinase		–1
3 Glyceraldehyde 3-P dehydrogenase	2 NADH	*5
4 Phosphoglycerate kinase		2
5 Pyruvate kinase		2
6 Pyruvate dehydrogenase	2 NADH	5
7 Isocitrate dehydrogenase	2 NADH	5
8 α-Ketoglutarate dehydrogenase	2 NADH	5
9 Succinyl CoA synthetase/ nucleoside diphosphate kinase		2
10 Succinate dehydrogenase	2FADH$_2$	3
11 Malate dehydrogenase	2 NADH	5
TOTAL		32

* Assumes malate/aspartate shuttle is used (see opposite)
NB The total of 32 does not allow for the energy used to transport phosphate and glutamate (equivalent to 1 ATP) so true net yield is 31 ATP, see JG Salway, Metabolism at a Glance, 3rd ed pp 20–21, Blackwell Publishing for full details

Figure 16.1 Aerobic oxidation of glucose to generate 32 molecules of ATP.

Malate/aspartate shuttle and glycerol 3-phosphate shuttle

How does NADH cross the mitochondrial inner membrane? The NADH produced by glyceraldehyde 3-phosphate dehydrogenase must enter the mitochondrion before it can be used to produce ATP. Problem: the inner membrane of the mitochondrial membrane is impermeable to NADH. The problem is overcome by processes that transfer the electrons (and protons) from NADH to malate or glycerol 3-phosphate, namely the **malate/aspartate shuttle** or the **glycerol 3-phosphate shuttle** (Fig. 16.2).

Malate/aspartate shuttle

Cytosolic malate dehydrogenase transfers the electrons and protons from **NADH** to **oxaloacetate** forming **malate**. Malate enters the mitochondrion via the **dicarboxylate carrier** in exchange for

α-ketoglutarate. **Mitochondrial malate dehydrogenase** transfers the electrons and protons to NAD^+ forming **oxaloacetate** and **NADH** which generates **2.5 molecules of ATP** in the respiratory chain. To complete the cycle, **oxaloacetate** is transaminated to **aspartate**, which enters the cytosol and is converted back to oxaloacetate.

Glycerol 3-phosphate shuttle

Cytosolic glyceraldehyde 3-phosphate dehydrogenase transfers the electrons and protons from **NADH** to **dihydroxyacetone phosphate**, forming **glycerol 3-phosphate**. **Mitochondrial glycerol 3-phosphate dehydrogenase** in the inner membrane transfers electrons and protons to its prosthetic group **FAD**, forming **FADH₂**, which passes to the respiratory chain and generates **1.5 molecules of ATP**. This reaction also generates dihydroxyacetone phosphate which completes the cycle.

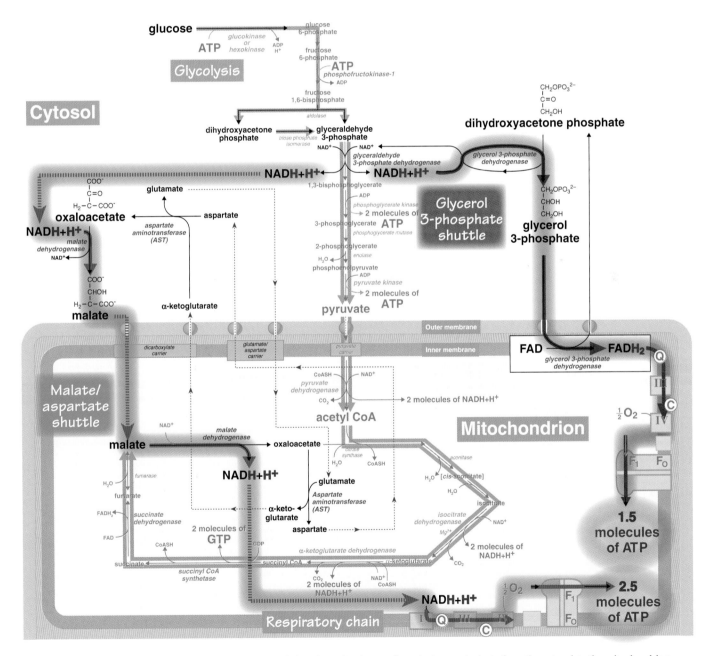

Figure 16.2 The malate/aspartate shuttle and the 3-glycerol phosphate shuttle transfer reducing equivalents from the cytosol to the mitochondrion.

Anaerobic oxidation of glucose by glycolysis to form ATP and lactate

17

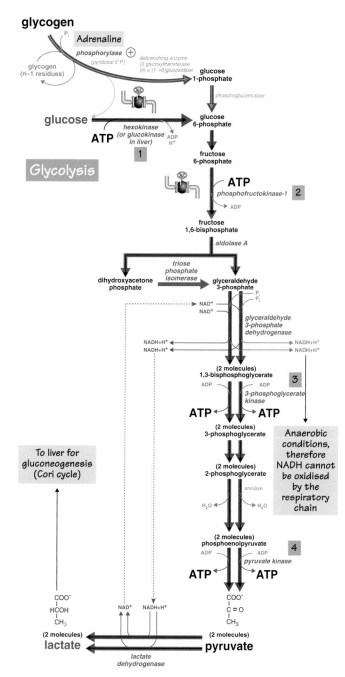

Figure 17.1 Anaerobic metabolism of glucose and glycogen to generate ATP.

Anaerobic glycolysis

Glucose can be metabolised to generate a **net total of two molecules of ATP** in the absence of oxygen, i.e. **anaerobically** (Fig. 17.1). As shown in Table 17.1, this initially needs the **investment** of ATP for each of the **hexokinase** and **phosphofructokinase** reactions. **Fructose 6-phosphate** is eventually split into **two molecules** of **glyceraldehyde 3-phosphate**, which when oxidised by **glyceraldehyde 3-phosphate dehydrogenase** yields **2 NADH**. **Two molecules** of **ATP** are produced by **3-phosphoglycerate kinase** and another **two molecules** of **ATP** are made in the **pyruvate kinase** reaction. *NB Under aerobic conditions, NADH is oxidised by the respiratory chain to recycle NAD⁺ for the glyceraldehyde 3-phosphate dehydrogenase reaction. (Remember that NAD⁺ and NADH are present in small amounts and must always be recycled.)* However, under **anaerobic** conditions **lactate dehydrogenase** causes NADH to reduce pyruvate and NAD⁺ is recycled for **glyceraldehyde 3-phosphate dehydrogenase**. The lactate goes to the liver and forms glucose by gluconeogenesis in the **Cori cycle** (Fig. 17.2).

Note that when glycogen is the source of glucose 6-phosphate, the net yield is **three molecules of ATP** (Table 17.2).

Table 17.1 Anaerobic glycolysis from glucose yields two molecules of ATP.

Yield of ATP from the anaerobic oxidation of glucose to lactate		
Reaction	NADH or FADH$_2$	ATP yield
1 Hexokinase (or glucokinase in liver)		−1
2 Phosphofructokinase-1		−1
3 3-Phosphoglycerate kinase		2
4 Pyruvate kinase		2
	TOTAL	2

Table 17.2 Anaerobic glycolysis from glycogen yields three molecules of ATP.

Yield of ATP from the anaerobic oxidation of a glucose residue derived from glycogen to lactate		
Reaction	NADH or FADH$_2$	ATP yield
2 Phosphofructokinase-1		−1
3 3-Phosphoglycerate kinase		2
4 Pyruvate kinase		2
	TOTAL	3

 Medical Biochemistry at a Glance, Third Edition. J. G. Salway. © 2012 John Wiley & Sons, Ltd. Published 2012 by John Wiley & Sons, Ltd.

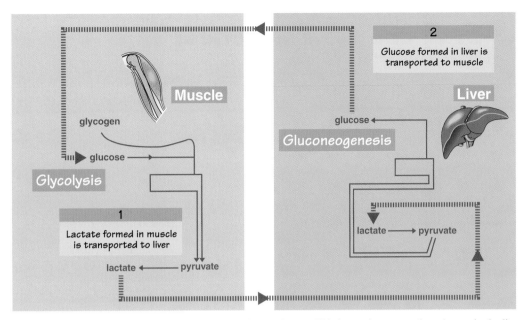

Figure 17.2 The Cori cycle. Glucose consumed by the liver is metabolised to lactate. This lactate is converted to glucose in the liver and recycled to muscle.

Fate of the lactate: the Cori cycle

Lactate is being produced continuously from glucose by anaerobic glycolysis in red blood cells, the retina and the kidney medulla. This lactate is recycled to glucose by a process known as the Cori cycle. The lactate is returned to the liver and is metabolised to glucose by **gluconeogenesis** in a process that consumes the equivalent of six molecules of ATP (Chapter 34). If the Cori cycle is interrupted by liver disease, lactate accumulates resulting in hyperlactataemia. Asymptomatic hyperlactataemia is a benign condition that is fairly common and rarely progresses to life-threatening lactic acidosis, which overwhelms the body's buffer systems.

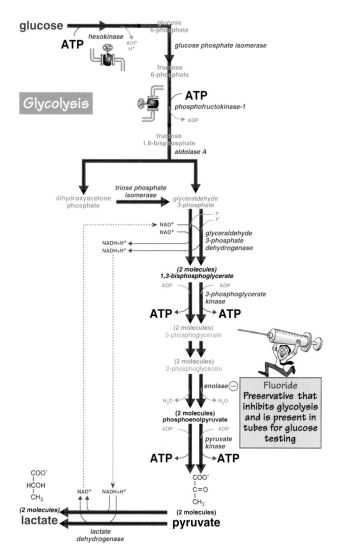

Figure 18.1 Anaerobic glycolysis in the red blood cell.

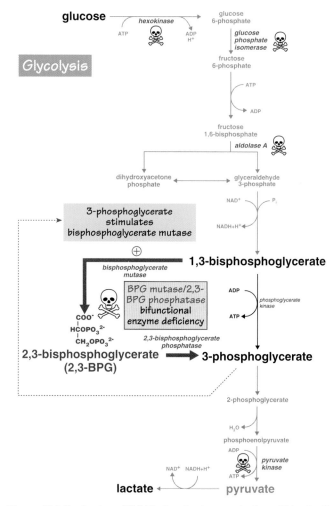

Figure 18.2 Production of 2,3-bisphosphoglycerate in the red blood cell.

The red blood cells contain an abundance of oxygen that they transport around the body, but ironically they cannot use this oxygen themselves and are entirely dependent on glucose for fuel by **anaerobic** glycolysis to produce ATP (Fig. 18.1). This is because they lack mitochondria and consequently the enzymes for the Krebs cycle. Similarly, red blood cells also lack the enzymes for fatty acid oxidation and ketone body utilisation.

The function of red blood cells is to transport oxygen, which they do by binding oxygen tightly to form **oxyhaemoglobin**. The problem is that when the red cells arrive at the peripheral tissue, they must be persuaded to unload their cargo of oxygen. They achieve this by the phenomenon known as the **Bohr effect**, which involves two contributing factors: **protons** and **2,3-bisphosphoglycerate** (**2,3-BPG**), as shown in Fig. 18.2.

1 Protons displace oxygen from oxyhaemoglobin. The production of ATP in exercising muscle involves the Krebs cycle, which produces **carbon dioxide** (CO_2). CO_2 enters the red cell where **carbonic anhy-**

drase catalyses its reaction with water to form **carbonic acid**. Carbonic acid decomposes spontaneously to **bicarbonate** and results in a localised **increase in the concentration of protons [H^+]** (i.e. a decrease in pH). These protons release oxygen from haemoglobin. The oxygen then diffuses from the red cell into the peripheral tissues where it binds to myoglobin, which transports the oxygen to the respiratory chain where it is used to produce ATP by oxidative phosphorylation. (The carbonic anhydrase reaction is described in a different context in Chapters 3–5.)

2 Unloading oxygen in the periphery: 2,3-BPG. The other factor that displaces oxygen from oxyhaemoglobin is 2,3-BPG (Fig. 18.2). This is better known in clinical circles as **2,3-diphosphoglycerate** (**2,3-DPG**). The 2,3-BPG is formed under anoxic conditions in red blood cells by the 2,3-BPG shunt (**Rapoport–Luebering shunt**) (Fig. 18.2). In the peripheral tissues, a molecule of 2,3-BPG binds to **deoxyhaemoglobin** which stabilises the structure and prevents it from grabbing hold of oxygen from adjacent molecules of **oxyhaemoglobin**.

3 Loading oxygen in the lungs. The red blood cells transport **deoxyhaemoglobin** and its cargo of CO_2 to the lungs. In the lungs there is a high partial pressure of oxygen that displaces the CO_2, which is exhaled from the lungs. Now oxygen binds to form **oxyhaemoglobin**, 2,3-BPG is displaced and the red cell proceeds to the periphery with its new load of oxygen.

2,3-BPG in health and disease
Fetal haemoglobin has a low affinity for 2,3-BPG
Haemoglobin is a tetramer of two α-chains and two β-chains. However, fetal haemoglobin consists of two α-chains and two γ-chains. Fetal haemoglobin has a lower affinity for 2,3-BPG than adult haemoglobin. This means that fetal haemoglobin has an affinity for oxygen that is greater than the maternal haemoglobin and this facilitates oxygen transfer from the mother to the fetus.

2,3-BPG and adaptation to high altitudes
Anyone who lives at low altitude who has flown to a high-altitude location knows that even moderate exertion can cause breathlessness. Within a few days, adaptation occurs as the concentration of 2,3-BPG in the red cells increases, enabling the tissues to obtain oxygen despite its relatively diminished availability in the thin mountain air.

Increased 2,3-BPG is the body's response to a lack of oxygen
The concentration of 2,3-BPG is increased in smokers, which compensates for a diminished oxygen supply because of their chronic exposure to carbon monoxide. Also, a compensatory increase in 2,3-BPG is commonly seen in patients with chronic anaemia, obstructive lung disease, congenital heart disease and cystic fibrosis.

Red cell enzymopathies of the glycolytic pathway
Inherited diseases due to deficiency of red cell glycolytic enzymes are rare causes of hereditary, non-spherocytic haemolytic anaemia. This can be serious for two reasons as the red cell is entirely dependent on glycolysis for the production of (i) ATP, and (ii) 2,3-BPG.

The effect on 2,3-BPG metabolism varies (Fig. 18.2). If the disorder is **proximal** to the **2,3-BPG shunt** (e.g. deficiencies of **hexokinase**, **phosphoglucose isomerase** and **aldolase A**), the flow of metabolites through glycolysis will be decreased and consequently the concentration of 2,3-BPG will **fall**. If the deficiency is **distal** to the **2,3-BPG shunt** (e.g. **pyruvate kinase** deficiency), the concentration of 2,3-BPG will **rise**.

Finally, patients have been reported with deficiency of the bifunctional shunt enzyme, **BPG mutase/2,3-BPG phosphatase**, and these patients have low concentrations of 2,3-BPG.

Aldolase nomenclature
This can be confusing! Aldolase (full name: fructose 1,6-bisphosphate aldolase) is officially known as D-glyceraldehyde 3-phosphate lyase, EC 4.1.2.13). It has three functions:
1 It catalyses the condensation of dihydroxyacetone phosphate with glyceraldehyde 3-phosphate to form fructose 1,6-bisphosphate.
2 It catalyses the splitting of fructose 1,6-bisphosphate to dihydroxyacetone phosphate and glyceraldehyde 3-phosphate.
3 It catalyses the cleavage of structurally similar sugar phosphates, e.g. fructose 1-phosphate to dihydroxyacetone phosphate and glyceraldehyde (Chapter 22). (*NB This function was previously described as ketose phosphate 1-aldolase, EC 4.1.2.7.*)

In animals three forms of aldolase have been described:
1 **Aldolase A.** In blood a defective form of aldolase A is present in hereditary haemolytic anaemia (Fig. 18.2). Aldolase A also occurs in muscle.
2 **Aldolase B.** Deficiency of aldolase B causes hereditary fructose intolerance (Chapter 22). Aldolase B occurs in the liver, kidney and small intestine.
3 **Aldolase C.** Occurs in the brain.

19 Carbohydrates

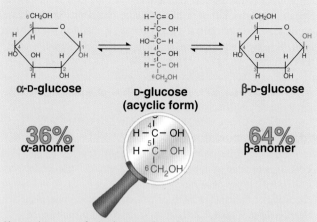

Nomenclature: confusion between D- and L-; d- and l-
The pioneers of carbohydrate chemistry used the "optical activity" (the ability to rotate the plane of polarised light clockwise or anticlockwise) to characterise carbohydrate structures. They observed that **glucose** and **fructose** rotated light to the **right** and **left** respectively and described them as "**d**" (**dextrorotatory**) and "**l**" (**laevorotatory**) (Latin: *dexter* right, and *laevus* left). Later, confusion arose when convention determined that the asymmetric atoms at C5 of **d-glucose** (and inconveniently **l-fructose!**) were configured in the D- convention (NB capital D) with the **OH group on the right-hand side of C5**. Therefore the terms "*d*" and "*l*" became obsolete and instead "+" and "-" were introduced to describe optical rotation

Glucose
The naturally occurring enantiomer of glucose is **D-glucose** also known by the arcane name **dextrose**. In medical circles confusion arises because glucose is often referred to as "**dextrose**" when it is infused into a patient, while the laboratory reports "**blood glucose**" concentrations. Even in medical literature, both dextrose and glucose are sometimes used in the same paper!

When glucose is dissolved in water, it has a structural identity crisis! It undergoes mutarotation and exists in ring forms or a straight chain. The two ring forms are 36% α-D-glucose or 64% β-D-glucose depending on the position of the OH group on the anomeric carbon atom, C1. If the OH group projects downwards, it is the **α-anomer**; if it projects upwards, it is the **β-anomer**. The **acyclic** ("straight chain") intermediate form comprises only 0.003% of the mixture.

Prolonged exposure of body proteins to high concentrations of glucose results in **glycation** which damages the proteins. This is known as "**glucose toxicity**" and is responsible for many of the complications of diabetes mellitus, Chapter 28

Figure 19.1 Carbohydrate nomenclature.

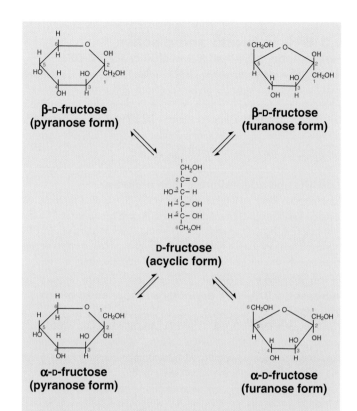

Naturally occurring D-**fructose** is also known by the arcane name, **laevulose**. Like glucose, fructose in solution also has an identity crisis: it exists in both α- and β- forms which in turn are changing between pyranose rings (6-membered rings) and furanose (5-membered rings). Fructose phosphates exist as furanose rings

Inulin. Several plants store a polymer of fructose called **inulin** (do not confuse with **insulin**) as a food reserve which is analogous to starch. Onions, leeks and bananas contain inulin but it is notoriously present in tubers of Jerusalem artichoke (*Helianthus tuberosus*). Since inulin is poorly digested it causes flatulence hence their irreverent nickname Jerusalem "Fartichokes". On a positive note, the "**inulin clearance test**" is the gold standard test for glomerular filtration since following intravenous infusion it is completely excreted in the urine

Figure 19.2 Structure of fructose.

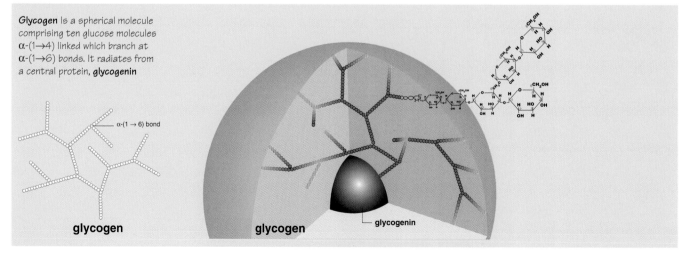

Glycogen Is a spherical molecule comprising ten glucose molecules α-(1→4) linked which branch at α-(1→6) bonds. It radiates from a central protein, **glycogenin**

Figure 19.3 Glycogen.

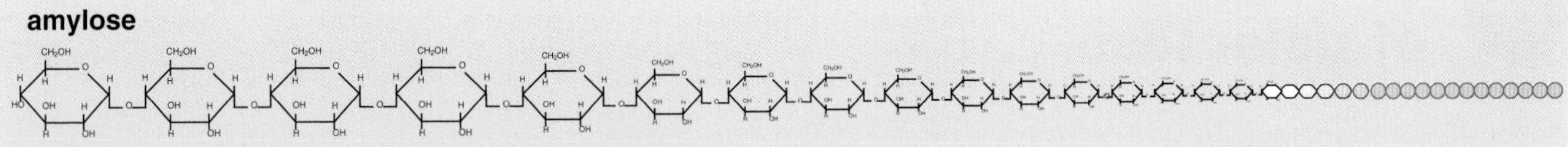

amylose

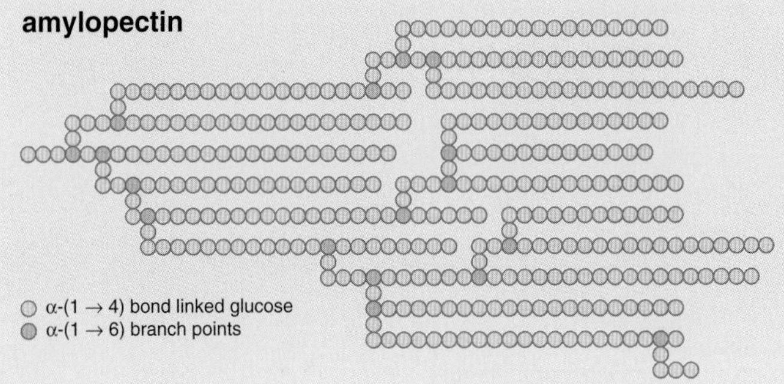

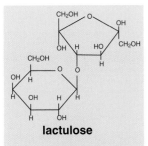

amylopectin

○ α-(1 → 4) bond linked glucose
● α-(1 → 6) branch points

Plants store carbohydrate mainly as starch. Starch is a polymer of glucose consisting of **amylose** (straight chain α-(1 → 4) linkages) and **amylopectin** (straight chains but with α-(1 → 6) bonds which cause branching). Dietary starch is digested by salivary α-amylase and pancreatic α-amylase producing **maltose** from the straight chains and **isomaltose** from the (1 → 6) linked glucose at the branch points

Figure 19.4 Starch.

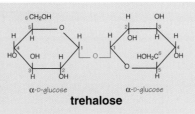

lactulose

This is a laxative and is a synthetic disaccharide comprising galactose and fructose. It is a stool softener, and since it is also a colonic acidifier, it removes ammonia from the blood in liver failure

Figure 19.5 Lactulose.

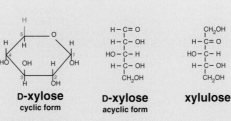

D-xylose cyclic form   **D-xylose** acyclic form   **xylulose**

D-Xylose occurs in grains and fruits. It is a pentose with a structure similar to its hexose cousin glucose. Since it is absorbed and excreted mainly unchanged, the **xylose tolerance test** is used to diagnose intestinal malabsorption syndromes.
NB **Xylose** is an aldose and **xylulose** is a ketose

Figure 19.6 D-xylose and xylulose.

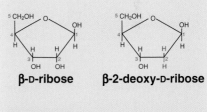

β-D-ribose   **β-2-deoxy-D-ribose**

Ribose is a pentose found in ribonucleic acid (RNA)
Deoxyribose, found in deoxyribonucleic acid (DNA), is derived from ribose by replacing the hydroxyl group at carbon 2 with hydrogen

Figure 19.7 Ribose and deoxyribose.

Trehalose occurs in the cocoons of the beetle Trehala manna and is thought to be the "**manna**" of biblical fame. The sweetness of mannose is due to **trehalose** (two glucose molecules joined by α-1 bonding). Trehalose is found in the haemolymph of insects and in mushrooms. Trehalose **stabilises the tertiary structure of proteins** (Chapter 8) enabling them to resist denaturation when subjected to dehydration. For example, the "Resurrection plant" or "Rose of Jericho" (Selaginella lepidophylla) which contains trehalose can withstand total drought for several years and when soaked with water will uncurl and flourish. This property of trehalose is used to store proteins such as hormones and antibodies

Preservation of vaccines using trehalose
A big problem with vaccines is storage. From the place of manufacture, through storage and transport to the doctor's clinic, they must be kept chilled or frozen. If they become warm, their efficacy is lost. In wealthy countries this logistical "cold-chain" is a costly inconvenience. In poor countries with a hot climate, the cold-chain does not exist. In 2010 scientists at Oxford University reported that vaccines, when stabilised with trehalose and sucrose, can be dehydrated and transported at ambient temperatures. It is envisaged that vaccines could be taken to remote villages in a bag strapped to a bicycle

α-D-glucose   α-D-glucose
trehalose

Figure 19.8 Trehalose.

---

sorbitol   **mannitol**   **galactitol**   **xylitol**

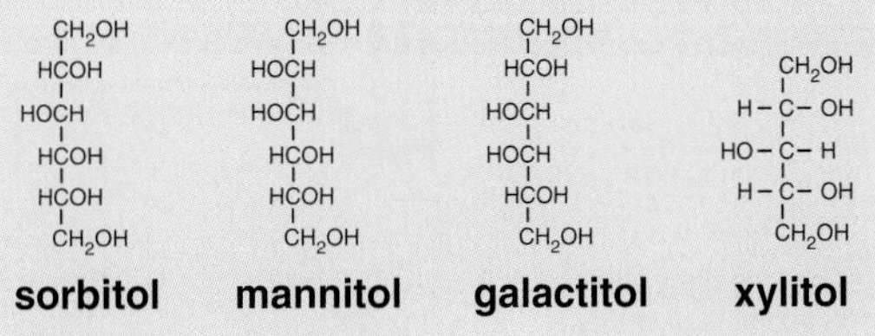

The **sugar alcohols** are polyols
Sorbitol was used by diabetic patients as a bulk sweetener. However, it is now considered to be of no benefit.
Intravenous **mannitol** is used as a diuretic.
Galactitol accumulates in people with galactosaemia.
Xylitol is the sugar alcohol form of xylose. It is extracted from birch wood and is also called "wood sugar". Xylitol is used as an anticariogenic sweetener in chewing gum

Figure 19.9 Sugar alcohols.

20

Absorption of carbohydrates and metabolism of galactose

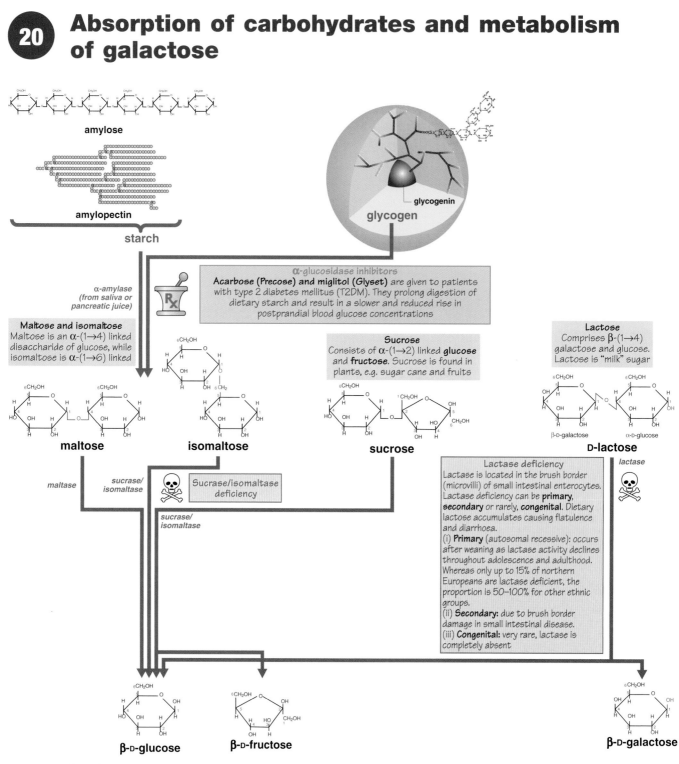

Figure 20.1 Absorption of carbohydrates.

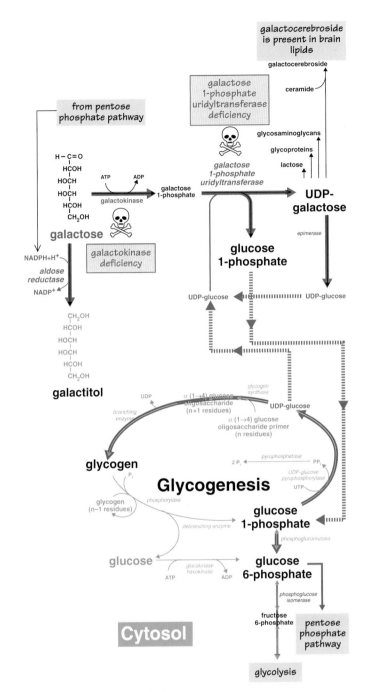

Figure 20.2 Galactose metabolism.

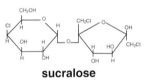

Galactose metabolism

The main dietary source of galactose is the disaccharide it forms with glucose, namely lactose (Fig. 20.1). **Lactose** (milk sugar) is hydrolysed in the intestine by **lactase**, and the **glucose** and **galactose** produced are transported directly to the liver via the hepatic portal vein. Galactose can enter the pathways used for glucose metabolism as follows. It is phosphorylated by **galactokinase** to galactose 1-phosphate (Fig. 20.2). Galactose 1-phosphate in the presence of **galactose 1-phosphate uridyltransferase (Gal-1-PUT)** forms **glucose 1-phosphate**. Gal-1-PUT also forms **uridine diphosphate (UDP) galactose** which can also be metabolised to **glucose 1-phosphate** by **epimerase**. The glucose 1-phosphate can be metabolised to glycogen, or to glucose 6-phosphate and then via glycolysis or the pentose phosphate pathway.

Galactose metabolism in disease

Galactose 1-phosphate uridyltransferase deficiency (Gal-1-PUT deficiency) is a rare autosomal recessive disorder that results in galactosaemia and galactosuria. It is usually manifest shortly after birth when the baby has feeding difficulties, with vomiting and failure to thrive. If not treated, liver damage, mental retardation and formation of cataracts can result.

A disease with similar symptoms occurs in **galactokinase** deficiency. In both cases, galactose accumulates and it is reduced to galactitol by aldose reductase.

Treatment is achieved by avoiding galactose and lactose in the diet. *(NB Do not confuse these conditions with **lactose intolerance** associated with **lactase deficiency**; Fig. 20.1.)*

Figure 20.3 Sucralose is a sweetener made from sucrose by substituting three chlorine atoms for three hydroxyl groups. It is claimed to be poorly absorbed and not metabolised.

Fate of glucose in liver: glycogenesis and lipogenesis

21

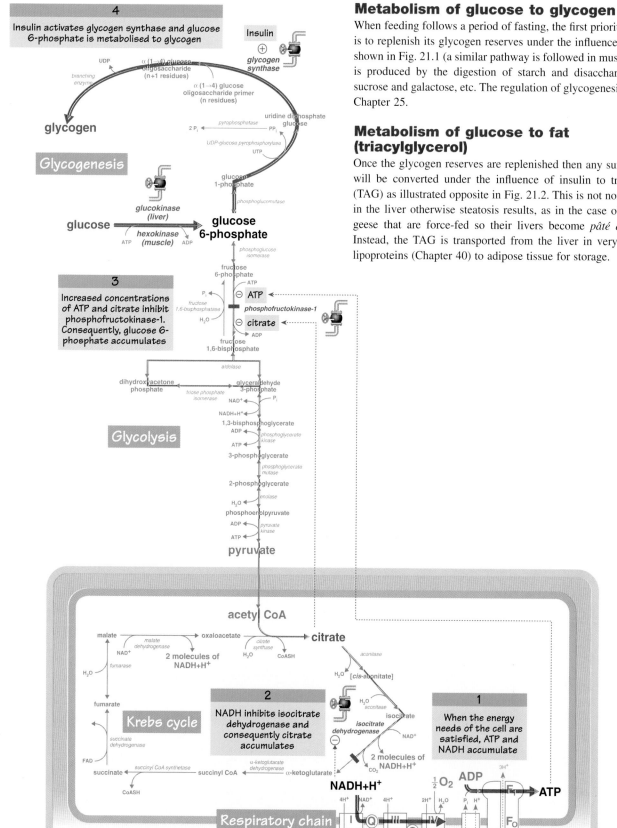

Metabolism of glucose to glycogen

When feeding follows a period of fasting, the first priority of the liver is to replenish its glycogen reserves under the influence of insulin as shown in Fig. 21.1 (a similar pathway is followed in muscle). Glucose is produced by the digestion of starch and disaccharides such as sucrose and galactose, etc. The regulation of glycogenesis is shown in Chapter 25.

Metabolism of glucose to fat (triacylglycerol)

Once the glycogen reserves are replenished then any surplus glucose will be converted under the influence of insulin to triacylglycerol (TAG) as illustrated opposite in Fig. 21.2. This is not normally stored in the liver otherwise steatosis results, as in the case of unfortunate geese that are force-fed so their livers become *pâté de foie gras*. Instead, the TAG is transported from the liver in very low density lipoproteins (Chapter 40) to adipose tissue for storage.

Figure 21.1 Metabolism of glucose to glycogen in liver.

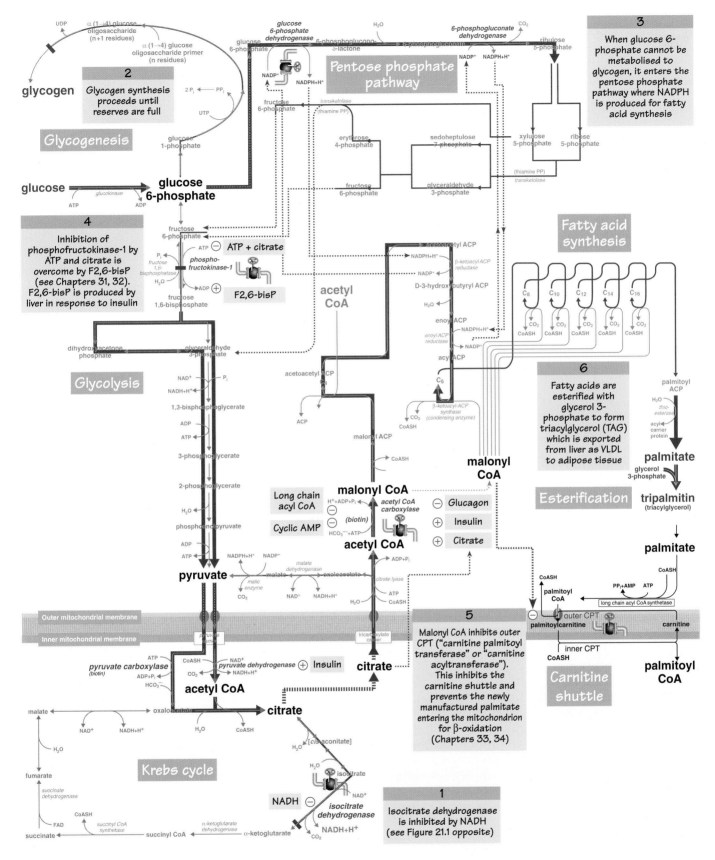

Figure 21.2 Metabolism of glucose to fatty acids and triacylglycerol (TAG) in liver.

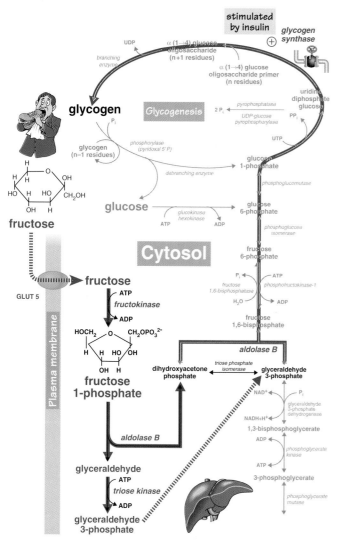

Figure 22.1 Fructose metabolism in liver.

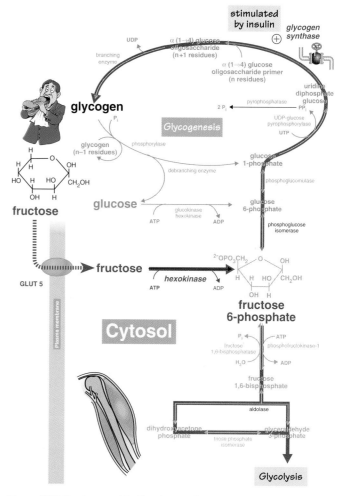

Figure 22.2 Fructose metabolism in muscle.

Fructose metabolism
Fructose metabolism in liver

Fructose is "fruit sugar" and, as its name implies, it is present in fruit. It is also, in combination with glucose, a component of the disaccharide, sucrose (table sugar), which is hydrolysed in the intestines by sucrase/isomaltase (Chapter 20). Thus, dietary fructose is transported from the intestine directly to the liver for metabolism as shown in Fig. 22.1. Fructose enters the liver cell by the inappropriately named "glucose transporter" **GLUT5**. It is then phosphorylated by **fructokinase** to form **fructose 1-phosphate** which is metabolised by **aldolase B** to **dihydroxyacetone phosphate** and **glyceraldehyde**. The latter is phosphorylated to **glyceraldehyde 3-phosphate** and both this and **dihydroxyacetone phosphate** enter glycolysis. In the fed state, it is probable that the fructose will be metabolised by the liver to glycogen and/or triacylglycerols. (NB "**aldolase**" also catalyses the reversible cleavage of fructose 1,6-bisphosphate to dihydroxyacetone phosphate and glyceraldehyde 3-phosphate; see "Aldolase nomenclature", Chapter 18.)

Fructose metabolism in muscle

Fructose metabolism in muscle is illustrated in Fig. 22.2. Fructose is phosphorylated by **hexokinase** to **fructose 6-phosphate**. The fructose 6-phosphate is then used for glycogenesis or, when the glycogen reserves are full, energy metabolism via glycolysis.

Fructose metabolism in disease
Fructokinase deficiency (essential fructosuria)

Hepatic fructokinase deficiency (Fig. 22.3) is a rare, benign disorder in which fructose accumulates in the blood and urine. It is most commonly found in Jewish families and subjects have a normal life expectancy. Sometimes the fructose in the urine is confused with glucose and this can lead to an incorrect diagnosis of diabetes mellitus.

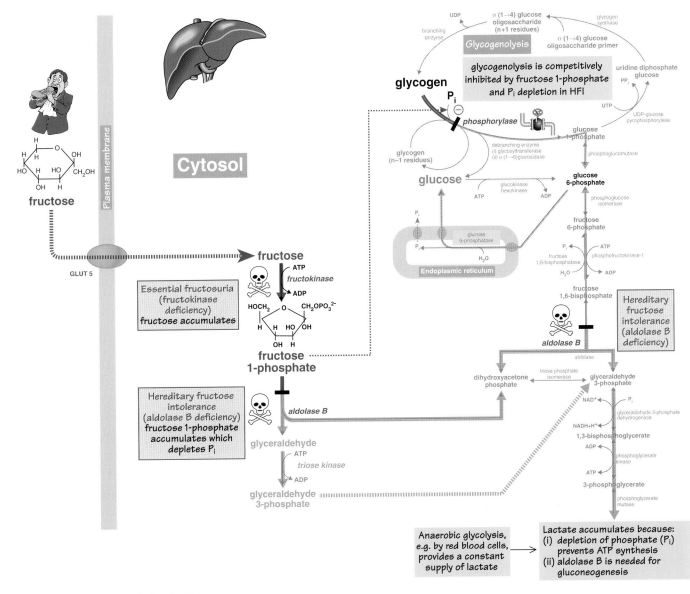

Figure 22.3 Fructose metabolism in disease.

Hereditary fructose intolerance (HFI) or aldolase B deficiency

HFI is an autosomal recessive disorder due to deficiency of the liver enzyme, **aldolase B** (Fig. 22.3). This serious condition is usually apparent when an infant is weaned from breast milk to food containing fructose. The response within 20 minutes of feeding is violent vomiting and hypoglycaemia. Lactic acid accumulates, causing metabolic acidosis with compensatory hyperventilation. If not treated, failure to thrive progresses to cachexia and continuing liver damage progresses to cirrhosis.

The pathology is due to accumulation of fructose 1-phosphate in liver following feeding with fructose-containing food. It almost immediately causes a log-jam of metabolites with gridlock particularly of glycogenolysis and gluconeogenesis, with collateral traffic chaos in adjacent pathways. Accumulation of fructose 1-phosphate has the following effects:

1 It depletes inorganic phosphate (Pi) thereby **inhibiting** both **glycogen phosphorylase** and the **synthesis of ATP**.
2 Inhibition of these reactions prevents hepatic glucose production resulting in **hypoglycaemia**.
3 Furthermore, **AMP accumulates** and is degraded to **urate** resulting in **hyperuricaemia** (Chapter 59).

The result is that liver metabolism effectively comes to a standstill. However, anaerobic metabolism elsewhere (e.g. by the red blood cells) continues to provide the liver with lactic acid which cannot be disposed of as usual by the Cori cycle (Chapter 17). The consequence is **lactic acidosis**.

Treatment simply involves avoiding dietary sources of fructose and compounds that are metabolised to fructose such as sucrose and sorbitol. Children develop a natural aversion to sweet foods and learn to avoid fructose. A positive outcome is that they are relatively free from dental caries.

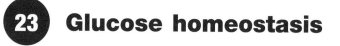

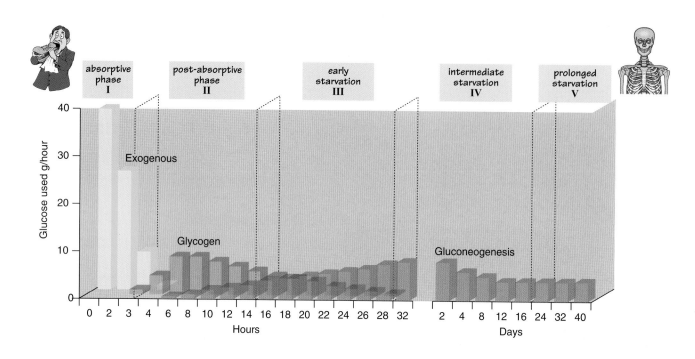

Figure 23.1 Rate of glucose utilisation during the five phases of glucose homeostasis. Adapted from Ruderman NB (1975) Muscle amino acid metabolism and gluconeogenesis. *Annu Rev Med* **26**, 245–58.

Importance of glucose homeostasis

The fasting blood glucose concentration is normally maintained between 3.5 and 5.5 mmol/l. After a meal, the blood glucose concentration normally rises briefly above 5.5 mmol/l, up to about 9 mmol/l, but within 2 hours it will return to the fasting level. Conversely, it is a remarkable fact that the body normally is capable of maintaining the blood glucose concentration above 3.5 mmol/l despite the challenges of prolonged starvation or strenuous exercise. For example, glucose homeostasis is maintained despite the sudden massive demand for glucose made by an athletic sprinter or by a Marathon runner. If this did not happen, the blood glucose concentration would fall and the brain would be deprived of fuel. Result: death!

Prevention of hypoglycaemia: major concepts

1 The preferred fuel of the brain is glucose. If the blood glucose concentration falls (hypoglycaemia), the brain is deprived of fuel (neuroglycopenia) which progressively results in unconsciousness, coma, brain damage and inevitably death.

2 The immediate reserve of glucose is liver glycogen. This is mobilised by glucagon within a few hours of fasting to maintain the normal blood glucose concentration. (NB Muscle reserves glycogen for its own use.)

3 The brain cannot use fatty acids as a fuel. This is because they are transported in the blood bound to albumin, which is too big to cross the blood–brain barrier.

4 The brain uses ketone bodies as fuel. If starvation continues for more than 2 days the brain adapts to using the ketone bodies as a fuel. Remember, during fasting, the liver converts fatty acids to ketone bodies.

5 Muscles and other tissues are converted to glucose. During starvation, tissue proteins are broken down (tissue wasting) to form amino acids. The liver metabolises the "glucogenic" amino acids by gluconeogenesis to glucose (Chapter 46). The "ketogenic" amino acids are metabolised by the liver to form the ketone bodies, while some amino acids are both ketogenic and glucogenic.

6 Fatty acids cannot form glucose. During starvation, it is most unfortunate that **fatty acids cannot be metabolised to glucose**

(Chapter 34). This means that once the glycogen reserves are exhausted, the principal gluconeogenic precursors are amino acids which are derived from tissue breakdown.

Harmful effects of hyperglycaemia

In uncontrolled diabetes mellitus, the blood glucose concentration commonly rises to 20 mmol/l (hyperglycaemia) but, in extreme cases, blood glucose concentrations of up to 60 mmol/l are seen. Although glucose is an important metabolic fuel, an abnormally high blood glucose concentration is harmful for the following reasons:

1 Osmotic effect. High blood glucose concentrations significantly increase the osmotic pressure of the blood resulting in water diffusing from the cells, into the blood and being excreted by the kidneys. The result is that the tissues become dehydrated, and dehydration of the brain cells inevitably results in coma.

2 Protein glycation. Modest increases in the blood glucose concentration result in glucose reacting non-enzymically with the free amino groups of amino acid residues in cellular and extracellular proteins. They are associated with the development of the chronic complications associated with diabetes such as neuropathy, nephropathy and retinopathy (Chapter 28).

3 Formation of reactive oxygen species (ROS). Evidence suggests that hyperglycaemia results in the formation of ROS (Chapter 15). Because ROS damage lipids, protein and DNA, they are thought to contribute to the pathogenesis of diabetic complications.

Five phases of glucose homeostasis

Figure 23.1 illustrates the origin of blood glucose following a meal and then progressing to a 40-day fast. The origin of the blood glucose can be classified into five phases:

1 Absorptive phase I. When dietary (exogenous) carbohydrate is digested and absorbed, glucose is abundant and the blood glucose concentration tends to rise. Insulin is secreted from pancreatic β-cells. Liver and muscle metabolise glucose to glycogen. When the glycogen reserves are full, liver metabolises glucose to triacylglycerols which are transported as very low density lipoprotein (VLDL) to the adipose tissue for storage.

2 Post-absorptive phase II. After about 3 hours, the exogenous glucose will have been disposed of. The pancreatic α-cells secrete glucagon and this promotes the breakdown of liver glycogen, which contributes to the blood glucose concentration. Note that after about 6 hours, glucagon begins to stimulate the liver to perform gluconeogenesis.

3 Early starvation phase III. Approximately 14 hours after the meal (which approximates to the interval between an early evening dinner and a leisurely breakfast) the glucose being used is derived equally from glycogen and gluconeogenesis. Glucose derived from glycogen continues to decline whereas glucose derived from gluconeogenesis becomes more important until 32 hours of starvation.

4 Intermediate starvation phase IV. After 32 hours of starvation, the liver's glycogen reserves are exhausted. From now on, the only source of glucose is gluconeogenesis, which is produced under the influence of the glucocorticosteroid hormone, cortisol. Fortunately, since gluconeogenesis is associated with tissue wasting, the liver produces ketone bodies from fatty acids and the brain adapts to use ketone bodies as a fuel. This process spares glucose and helps to minimise the provision of gluconeogenic substrates by muscle wasting.

5 Prolonged starvation phase V. After about 16 days' starvation, an average person with access to water might survive another 24 days without food in phase V of glucose homeostasis (i.e. a total of 40 days). During this final phase, glucose is provided entirely by gluconeogenesis. The ketone bodies are now the major fuel of the brain, thereby sparing glucose, which is consumed by the brain at a diminished rate.

Gluconeogenesis, muscle wasting and failure of wound healing

Although glucagon begins to stimulate gluconeogenesis after about 6 hours of fasting, it is from 32 hours onwards when cortisol contributes to gluconeogenesis that it is maximally stimulated. *NB The glucocorticosteroid hormone* **cortisol** *is a catabolic steroid and is active in the breakdown of proteins in muscle and other tissues to form amino acids which are used as gluconeogenic precursors.* Obviously, muscle wasting is a desperate strategy to supply the brain with glucose for energy metabolism. This observation leads to the importance of nutritional support in patients who are recovering from surgery or major injury such as crush syndrome or severe burns. If the patient is not consuming sufficient food, then a catabolic state will prevail. The result is that muscle and tissue wasting will occur, contrary to the need for the patient to be in an anabolic state enabling repair of the wounds.

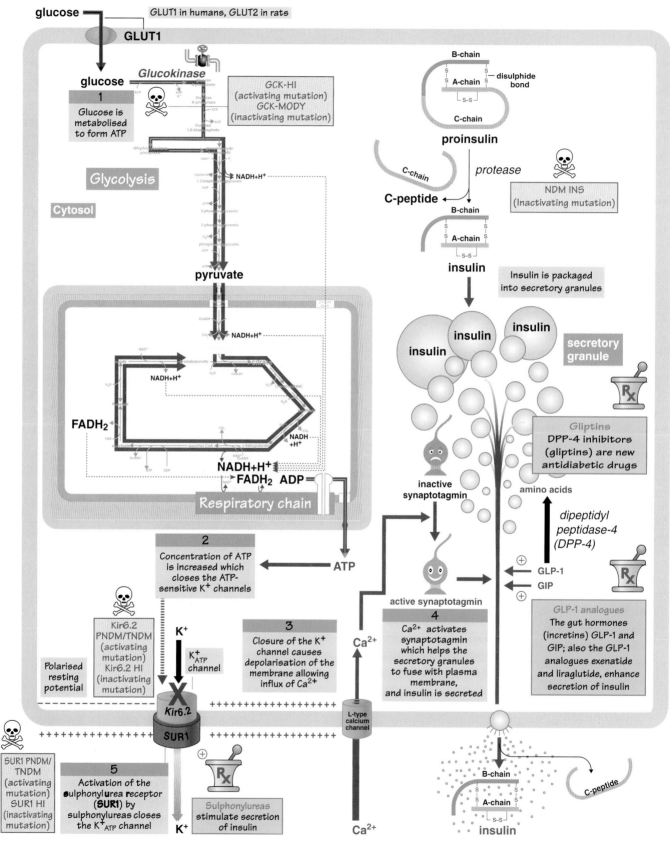

Figure 24.1 Metabolism of glucose produces ATP, which triggers insulin secretion from the pancreatic β-cells.

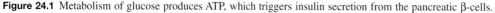

β-cell metabolism

The β-cells are the cells within the islets of Langerhans of the pancreas that manufacture, store and secrete insulin. Insulin is secreted after a meal and the metabolic fuel hypothesis proposes this is linked to the metabolism of glucose by the β-cells to produce ATP, and ATP is the biochemical signal that triggers insulin secretion. Thus, when increasing amounts of carbohydrate-containing food are absorbed, then increasing amounts of glucose will be metabolised to ATP and this will trigger proportionate amounts of insulin to be secreted.

The several steps in this process are summarised in Table 24.1 (the numbers relate to Fig. 24.1).

Incretins potentiate insulin secretion.

Incretins are the gut hormones, **GLP-1** (glucagon-like peptide 1) and **GIP** (glucose-dependent insulinotropic polypeptide), which enhance the secretion of insulin in response to a meal (Fig. 24.1). GLP-1 has the potential to be a useful antidiabetic drug, but it is rapidly broken down by dipeptidyl peptidase 4 (DPP-4). To overcome this, GLP analogues (i.e. **incretin mimetics**) that are resistant to DPP-4 have been made, e.g. exenatide and liraglutide. Also, **DPP-4 inhibitors** (gliptins), which are **incretin enhancers**, have been introduced or are in clinical trials, e.g. sitagliptin, vidagliptin, saxagliptin and alogliptin.

Table 24.1 Metabolism of glucose produces ATP, which triggers insulin secretion from the pancreatic β-cells (Fig. 24.1).

---

1 Glucose enters the β-cell via the **GLUT1** glucose transporter (GLUT1 in humans, GLUT2 in rodents). It is then phosphorylated by **glucokinase** prior to being metabolised by **glycolysis**, **Krebs cycle** and the **respiratory chain** to produce **ATP**
2 The change in the ratio of **ATP to ADP due to the increased ATP from glucose metabolism closes the ATP-sensitive potassium channels** (K_{ATP} channels)
3 At rest, the plasma membrane is polarised. It has a resting potential with the inside of the membrane having a negative charge. When the **potassium channels are closed by ATP, K^+ ions (positively charged) accumulate** and neutralise the negative charges on the inside surface of the membrane thus **depolarising the membrane**. Depolarisation activates calcium channels causing an **influx of Ca^{2+} ions**
4 Ca^{2+} ions **activate synaptotagmin**, which helps the secretory granules containing insulin to fuse with the plasma membrane and insulin is secreted
5 Kir6.2/SUR1 complex. The **sulphonylurea** drugs (e.g. glibenclamide, gliclazide, tolbutamide) bind to **SUR1** (sulphonylurea receptor) causing it to close the K_{ATP} channels (Kir6.2), which depolarises **the membrane and promotes insulin secretion**

Inborn errors of β-cell metabolism can cause excessive or insufficient production of insulin

These are rare inborn errors that result in **hypo**glycaemia or **hyperg**lycaemia, respectively.

Excessive production of insulin

Inappropriate hypersecretion of insulin causes **hyperinsulinism** (**HI**). There are a number of causes of HI but the most common are due to **inactivating** mutations in **the K_{ATP} channel genes** (*KCNJ11* and *ABCC8*) which encode **Kir6.2** and **SUR1**, respectively. HI can also be caused by **activating** mutations in the **glucokinase** (*GCK*) gene (Table 24.2 and Fig. 24.1).

Insufficient production of insulin

Maturity-**o**nset **d**iabetes of the **y**oung (**MODY**) is an autosomal dominantly inherited form of diabetes typically diagnosed before the age of 25 years that is characterised by β-cell dysfunction. There are a number of MODY subtypes caused by mutations in different β-cell genes. The two most common subtypes in the UK are **GCK-MODY** due to inactivating *GCK* mutations and **HNF1A-MODY** due to inactivating mutations in a key transcription factor regulating insulin synthesis and secretion (HNF1A or **h**epatocyte **n**uclear **f**actor 1 **a**lpha; gene name *HNF1A*).

Neonatal **d**iabetes **m**ellitus (**NDM**) is diagnosed within the first 6 months of life. NDM can either be **t**ransient (**TNDM**) or **p**ermanent (**PNDM**). The most common cause of TNDM is an abnormality of an imprinted region on chromosome 6p24. There are a number of genetic causes of PNDM but the most common causes are due to heterozygous activating mutations in *KCNJ11* and *ABCC8* and inactivating mutations in the insulin (*INS*) gene. Patients with NDM require treatment with insulin. However, it is now known that patients with NDM due to mutations in *KCNJ11* or *ABCC8* can be treated with sulphonylureas, which close the K_{ATP} channel by an ATP-independent mechanism and restore insulin secretion (Table 24.2 and Fig. 24.1).

Structure of the insulin molecule

Proinsulin is stored in the β-cells. It is converted to insulin in the secretory granules by proteases. Proteolytic cleavage of the C-chain produces active insulin, i.e. a dimer of the A- and B-chains (Fig. 24.1).

Table 24.2 Inborn errors of β-cell metabolism.

Glucokinase: heterozygous, activating mutation	**Glucokinase (GCK)** is **more active** causing inappropriately high β-cell glucose metabolism resulting in inappropriate insulin secretion causing **hyperinsulinaemia (GCK-HI)**
Glucokinase: heterozygous, inactivating mutation	Glucokinase is **less active** causing decreased β-cell glucose metabolism resulting in decreased insulin secretion and **maturity-onset diabetes of the young (GCK-MODY)**
Kir6.2: heterozygous, activating mutation (K inwardly rectifying channel)	K_{ATP} channels are **constantly open** which prevents insulin secretion and causes both **permanent** and **transient neonatal diabetes mellitus (Kir6.2-PNDM/TNDM)**
Kir6.2: heterozygous, inactivating mutation	K_{ATP} channels are **constantly inactive** (closed) which triggers constant insulin secretion causing **hyperinsulinaemia (Kir6.2-HI)**
SUR1: heterozygous activating mutation (sulphonylurea receptor)	**Activating** mutations cause the K_{ATP} channel to remain **open** preventing insulin secretion causing both **SUR1-PNDM and SUR1-TNDM**
SUR1: heterozygous, inactivating mutation	The **inactivating** SUR1 mutation stimulates constant closure of the K_{ATP} channel causing constant insulin secretion and hyperinsulinaemia (**SUR1-HI**)
Insulin (INS): heterozygous inactivating mutation	The mutations **prevent** the formation of disulphide bonds preventing **normal folding of proinsulin** in the endoplasmic reticulum (ER) leading to ER stress, β-cell apoptosis and neonatal diabetes mellitus (**INS-NDM**)
Hepatocyte nuclear factor 1 alpha (HNF1A): heterozygous inactivating mutation	Inactivating mutations **cause decreased transcriptional activity** influencing both pancreatic development and the transcription of key genes for insulin secretion (**HNF1A-MODY**)

25 Regulation of glycogen metabolism

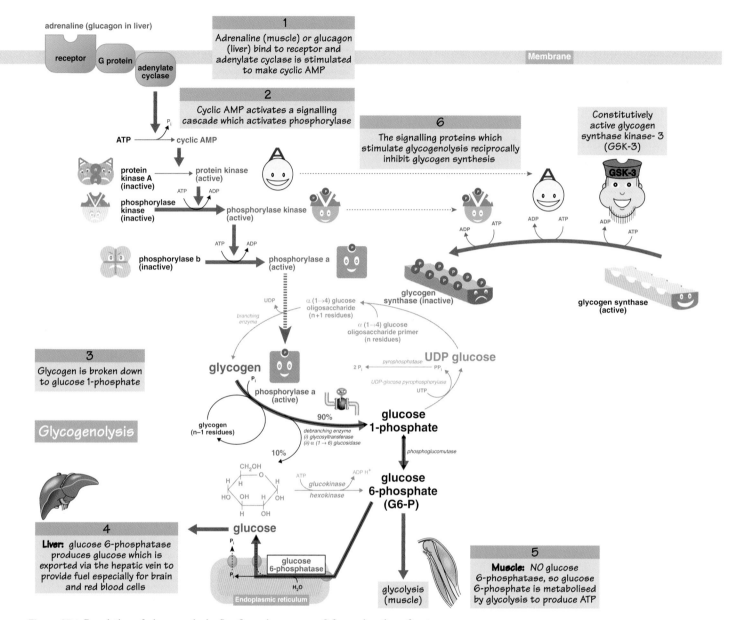

Figure 25.1 Regulation of glycogenolysis. See figure key on page 8 for explanation of cartoons.

Regulation of glycogenolysis (glycogen breakdown)

Glycogen is stored mainly in liver and muscle. The **liver** (the great provider) breaks down glycogen during periods of fasting to top up the blood glucose concentration for use as fuel by the brain and red blood cells. On the other hand, **muscle** (the fuel guzzler) uses glycogen for its own energy needs, especially for anaerobic glycolysis in a "flight or fight" emergency. In **muscle**, **adrenaline** initiates glycogenolysis by binding to its receptor and stimulating **adenylate cyclase** to produce **cyclic adenosine monophosphate** (AMP) (Fig. 25.1). Cyclic AMP activates a cascade of reactions that finally activates

phosphorylase causing glycogen breakdown. In the **liver**, **glucagon**, which is released from pancreatic α-cells during fasting, initiates glycogenolysis.

Regulation of glycogenesis (glycogen synthesis)

During feeding, both liver (Fig. 21.1) and muscle remove glucose from the blood and convert it to **glycogen**. Liver can also make fat (triacylglycerol) from glucose (Fig. 21.2). Glycogen synthesis is initiated when **insulin** binds to its **receptor**. This causes autophosphorylation of tyrosine residues in the insulin receptor, which triggers a chain of

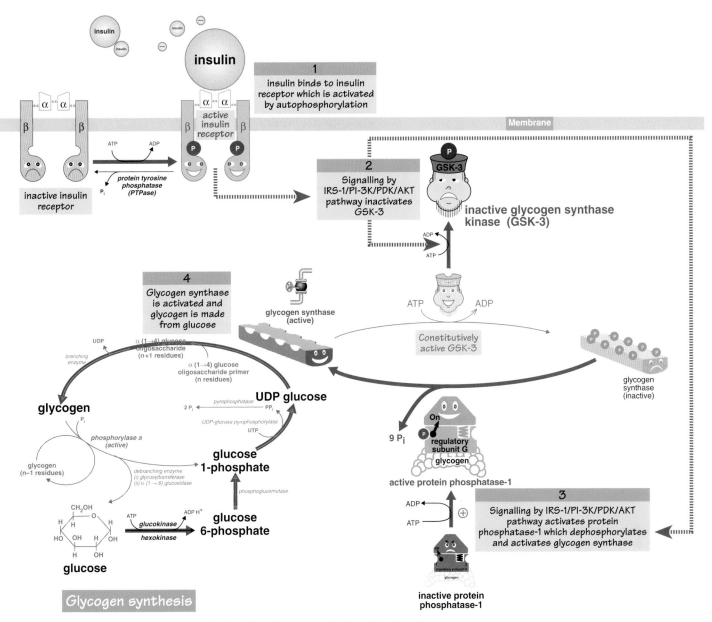

Figure 25.2 Regulation of glycogen synthesis. See figure key on page 8 for explanation of cartoons.

signalling proteins (**IRS-1/PI-3 kinase/PDK/AKT**; Chapter 27), which inactivates **glycogen synthase kinase 3** (**GSK-3**). During **fasting**, GSK-3 is constitutively **active**. In other words, it is only **inactive** after **feeding** in response to insulin signalling. As such, during fasting, **active GSK-3** applies the brakes to glycogen synthesis by phosphorylating and thus inactivating **glycogen synthase**. When insulin renders **GSK-3 inactive**, the signalling pathway **activates protein phosphatase 1** which dephosphorylates and **activates glycogen synthase**. Glycogen synthesis from glucose can now proceed.

Protein tyrosine phosphatase (PTPase) and PTPase inhibitors

Once feeding is finished, the insulin signal is terminated by dephosphorylating the tyrosine residues of the insulin receptor using PTPase. In a subgroup of patients with type 2 diabetes, PTPase is inappropriately active which results in attenuation of the insulin signal causing insulin resistance. Current research to discover PTPase inhibitors promises a novel treatment for type 2 diabetes.

26 Glycogen breakdown (glycogenolysis) and glycogen storage diseases

Glycogenolysis in health

Glycogen is stored in muscle and liver (Figs 26.1 and 26.2). It is mobilised in liver during starvation and in muscle during extreme exercise.

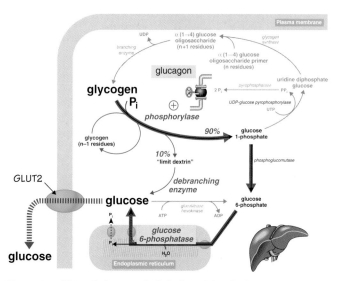

Figure 26.1 Normal glycogenolysis in liver. Liver is the "great provider" and during fasting (when glucagon prevails) its reserves of glycogen are broken down to release glucose into the blood where it is transported to the brain for energy metabolism. To achieve this, the **liver has glucose 6-phosphatase activity**.

Glycogen storage diseases (GSD)

The 12 glycogen storage diseases are characterised by abnormal accumulation of glycogen. Four examples are shown in Figs 26.3–26.6.

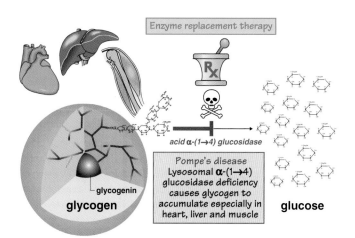

Figure 26.3 GSD II, Pompe's disease. GSD II (autosomal recessive) is caused by a deficiency of acid α-(1 → 4) glucosidase, a lysosomal enzyme. Glycogen accumulates, causing cardiomegaly after 2–3 months. The liver and muscle are also affected, causing generalised muscle weakness. Enzyme replacement therapy has been successful in Pompe's disease especially by reversing the pathology in cardiac muscle.

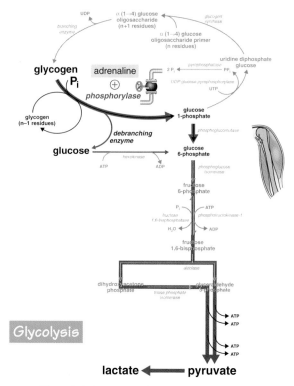

Figure 26.2 Normal glycogenolysis in muscle. Muscle, especially white skeletal muscle, uses glycogen entirely for its own benefit as a fuel especially during vigorous anaerobic exercise, e.g. during adrenaline-stimulated flight or fight. **Muscle does not have glucose 6-phosphatase activity**.

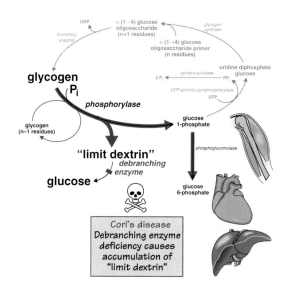

Figure 26.4 GSD III, Cori's disease. This is named after husband and wife, Carl and Gerty Cori (so note the apostrophe if you prefer "Coris's" disease). GSD III is caused by a deficiency of **debranching enzyme** so "**limit dextrin**" accumulates, which is an abnormal form of glycogen where the branches are reduced to α-(1→6) stumps. GSD III presents with hypoglycaemia and hepatomegaly.

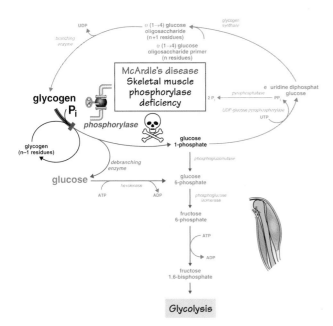

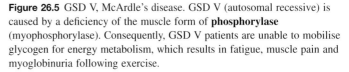

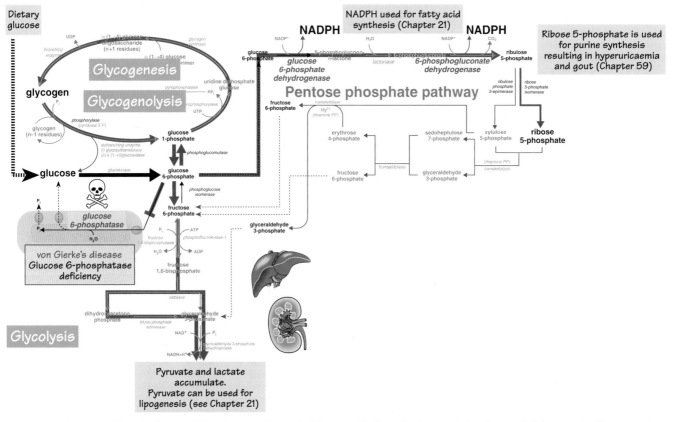

Figure 26.5 GSD V, McArdle's disease. GSD V (autosomal recessive) is caused by a deficiency of the muscle form of **phosphorylase** (myophosphorylase). Consequently, GSD V patients are unable to mobilise glycogen for energy metabolism, which results in fatigue, muscle pain and myoglobinuria following exercise.

Figure 26.6 GSD I, von Gierke's disease. GSD I (autosomal recessive) is caused by **hepatic glucose 6-phosphatase** deficiency so the liver loses its ability to prevent hypoglycaemia. Neonatal hypoglycaemia can be severe and glycogen is stored in excess in the liver and kidney. Other features that are a consequence of accumulation of glucose 6-phosphate are hyperlactataemia, hyperlipidaemia, hyperuricaemia and gout.

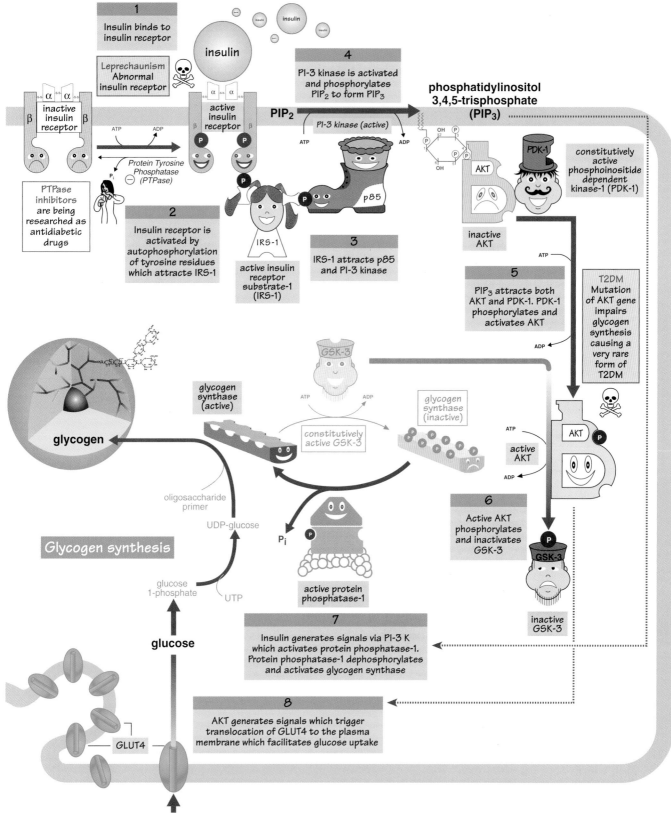

Figure 27.1 How insulin signal transduction stimulates glycogen synthesis (PDK/AKT hypothesis). See figure key on page 8 for explanation of cartoons.

Regulation of enzyme activity by reversible protein phosphorylation

Approximately one-third of cellular proteins contain phosphate and are subject to covalent modification by **phosphorylation** and **dephosphorylation** reactions. This reversible phosphorylation of proteins causes conformational changes in the protein that dramatically alters their properties, e.g. from an active to an inactive enzyme, or vice versa. The sites of protein phosphorylation are those amino acid residues that contain hydroxyl groups, most commonly **serine** but also **tyrosine** and **threonine** (Fig. 27.2) (Chapter 31). Phosphorylation uses **protein kinase** and dephosphorylation uses **protein phosphatase**. The importance of reversible protein phosphorylation to the living cell is emphasised by the fact that protein kinases and protein phosphatases comprise approximately 5% of the proteins encoded by the human genome. Current research is discovering abnormalities of protein phosphorylation that are associated with diseases, notably **type 2 diabetes mellitus** (**T2DM**) and cancer. In the future, the discovery of drugs that modify protein phosphorylation/dephosphorylation promises new therapies for the treatment of these diseases.

Insulin signal transduction: the PDK/AKT hypothesis

AKT was previously known as PKB. Insulin has scores of different effects on cells. It can stimulate the translocation of GLUT4 glucose transporters to the plasma membrane, and stimulate fatty acid synthesis, protein synthesis, glycogen synthesis, etc. Remarkably, all these effects are mediated though one insulin receptor and this phenomenon is known as the **pleiotropic** effects of insulin (pleiotropic is from the Greek, meaning "many ways"). The process begins with the binding of insulin to its receptor, which initiates a series of interactions between various signalling proteins, eventually resulting in an event that stimulates or inhibits a regulatory process.

In Fig. 27.1 we see how insulin binds to the insulin receptor. This activates tyrosine residues on the insulin receptor by the process of **autophosphorylation**. Once the insulin receptor is activated, it attracts and binds **insulin receptor substrate 1** (**IRS-1**). IRS-1 now attracts **p85** which is the regulatory subunit of PI-3 kinase. PI-3 kinase phosphorylates the 3 position of **phosphatidylinositol 4,5-bisphosphate** (**PIP$_2$**) to form **phosphatidylinositol 3,4,5-trisphosphate** (**PIP$_3$**). PIP$_3$ now attracts to the membrane **AKT** (previously known as **PKB**) and **PDK-1** so they are adjacent and **AKT** is activated by phosphorylation. AKT can now phosphorylate and inactivate **glycogen synthase kinase 3** (**GSK-3**). GSK-3 is constitutively active, and in the fasting state (i.e. in the absence of insulin) it phosphorylates and **inactivates glycogen synthase** which applies the brakes to the process of glycogen synthesis. So, we have now seen how insulin through AKT removes the inhibition by GSK-3 and **glycogen synthase is activated** following dephosphorylation by **protein phosphatase 1**. Meanwhile, another chain of signals mediated by AKT stimulates the translocation of **GLUT4** glucose transporters to the plasma membrane, which facilitates glucose uptake. The glucose can be metabolised to glycogen in the presence of active glycogen synthase.

Disorders of insulin signal transduction

Recent clinical research provides support for the validity of the PDK/AKT hypothesis and three examples are shown below.

Leprechaunism (Donohue's syndrome)

This is a very rare inborn error in which babies fail to thrive and have the features of mythical Irish elves know as "leprechauns". This causes severe diabetes and premature death. The insulin receptor is abnormal and cannot function adequately. This results in a failure of insulin signalling even though the β-cells of the pancreas are able to secrete insulin.

AKT (or PKB) mutation

A family has been described with a mutation of the gene that expresses AKT*. As predicted by the PDK/AKT hypothesis, this results in a very rare form of type 2 diabetes.

Protein tyrosine phosphatase

When feeding has finished, insulin secretion stops and insulin signal transduction within the cell must be terminated. Dephosphorylation of the insulin receptor by **protein tyrosine phosphatase** (**PTPase**) occurs, which inactivates the insulin receptor and insulin signalling ceases. However, there is evidence that some diabetic patients have a form of PTPase that is inappropriately active and opposes normal activation of the receptor by phosphorylation. Currently, there is a major research effort to develop drugs that inhibit PTPase and provide a new treatment for type 2 diabetes.

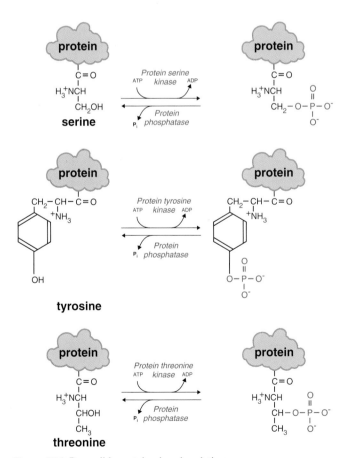

Figure 27.2 Reversible protein phosphorylation.

*George S, Rochford JJ, Wolfrum C *et al.* (2004) A family with severe insulin resistance and diabetes due to mutation in AKT2. *Science* **304**, 1325–8.

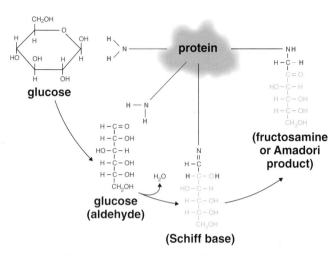

Figure 28.1 Glucose reacts non-enzymatically with free N-terminal α-amino groups and the ε-amino group of lysyl residues of proteins to form fructosamine products.

The term "diabetes" from the Greek *dia*, through, and *bainen*, to go, means "passing through" or "siphon" and describes the excessive production of urine (polyuria) in this condition. **Diabetes mellitus** (*mellitus*, honey) refers to the sweet taste of the urine, while in diabetes insipidus the urine is "insipid" (i.e. tasteless). (Don't worry, you don't have to taste the urine nowadays!) Diabetes is caused by **lack of insulin activity** while **diabetes insipidus** is caused by **insufficient vasopressin (antidiuretic hormone) activity**.

Diabetes mellitus (DM) is characterised by hyperglycaemia due to defective insulin secretion, defective insulin action or both. The global prevalence in 2010 is 285 million cases and this is projected to be 439 million in 2030. The main types are **type 1 DM** (T1DM) and **type 2 DM** (T2DM). There is also **gestational DM** and other unusual types such as **maturity-onset diabetes of the young (MODY)**.

Type 1 diabetes mellitus

T1DM was previously known as "insulin-dependent diabetes mellitus" (IDDM) and "juvenile-onset diabetes" (JOD). It occurs in 0.5% of the population, and is characterised by sudden onset, usually before 25 years of age, and weight loss. The **β-cells are destroyed by auto-immune attack** following viral infection. "Molecular mimicry" is thought to be the cause. This happens when parts of a virus protein resemble a protein in the host's β-cells. The body's immune defences then attack **both** the **virus** and the **β-cells**, which are destroyed: hence **insulin secretion ceases** causing T1DM.

Type 2 diabetes mellitus

T2DM was previously known as "non-insulin-dependent diabetes mellitus" (NIDDM) and "maturity-onset diabetes" (MOD). It occurs in 3–5% of the population, and typically is characterised by slow, insidious and progressive onset until diagnosis in middle age. T2DM is often associated with obesity.

The pathogenesis of T2DM has numerous causes. However, there is general agreement that T2DM involves a combination of **diminished insulin secretion from the β-cells** and **insulin resistance**.

Insulin resistance means that although insulin is present it does not work effectively. There are probably scores of explanations for why the insulin does not function, hence recent research suggests there are scores of different subtypes of T2DM. For example, insulin resistance could be caused by **structural abnormalities of any of the following**: the insulin molecule, the insulin receptor on the target tissue, the signalling proteins and enzymes involved in glucose and lipid uptake and metabolism (e.g. Chapters 21, 25, 27).

Gestational diabetes mellitus (GDM)

During pregnancy a transient period of insulin resistance is normal, but in about 4% of pregnancies insulin resistance is sufficiently severe to cause hyperglycaemia and GDM ensues. The cause of insulin resistance is not clear. However, **raised** levels of **oestrogen**, **human placental lactogen** and recently **low** levels of the insulin sensitiser, **adiponectin**, have been implicated.

Monogenic diabetes or maturity-onset diabetes of the young (MODY)

The term "maturity-onset diabetes of the young" was coined in 1974 when "maturity-onset diabetes" described what is now T2DM. MODY is currently being replaced with the nomenclature **monogenic diabetes**.

MODY occurs in approximately 1–2% of people with diabetes but often is diagnosed as either T1DM or T2DM. It is characterised by **early onset**. However, a difference from T1DM is that MODY patients are able to secrete insulin from the β-cells albeit at an insufficient rate or amount to control hyperglycaemia (Chapter 24). MODY is an inherited disorder with **autosomal dominant inheritance caused by a defect of a single gene**. There are at least six subtypes of MODY, which account for ~87% of cases in the UK. They are due to mutations in the genes encoding **glucokinase** (GCK-MODY) (Chapter 24) and the transcription factors **HNF4A, HNF1A, IPF1, HNF1B** and **NEUROD1**.

Glucose toxicity

Glucose is an important fuel for all tissues and is essential for red blood cells. Ironically, prolonged exposure of cells to **excessive concentrations of glucose can be harmful** through the following mechanisms.

Osmotic effects

The **hypertonic** effect of high glucose concentrations in the extracellular fluid causes **water** to be drawn **from cells into** the **extracellular fluid**, thence into the **blood** and **excretion** in the **urine**, resulting in **dehydration**.

β-cell damage caused by free radicals

High concentrations of glucose in β-cells result in **enhanced oxidative phosphorylation**, which generates increased amounts of reactive oxygen species (**ROS**) causing **oxidative stress** (Chapters 14, 15) and **loss of β-cell function**. The consequence is a reduced ability to secrete insulin, resulting in hyperglycaemia, and thus a **vicious cycle** of **hyperglycaemia/ROS/β-cell dysfunction** ensues **exacerbating** the **diabetes**.

Glycation of proteins

This describes the **non-enzymatic** reaction between **glucose** (and other reducing sugars) with free N-terminal α-amino groups or the ε-amino group of lysyl residues in proteins, which is a normal, but undesirable, ongoing process. **NB Although the reactant is glucose, the product is a fructosamine** (Fig. 28.1). Hyperglycaemia allows glucose to react with proteins in the plasma and tissues, resulting in the accumulation of **glycated products**. Over periods of months and years, these form **advanced glycation end products (AGEs)**, which **cross-link** long-lived proteins, e.g. **collagen**, resulting in dysfunction and the pathogenesis of **diabetic complications** such as vascular stiffening, hypertension, nephropathy and retinopathy.

*NB The nomenclature is confused for glycosylation and glycation. Over the past decades, the terminology has varied. However, the nomenclature currently in favour is: **glycosylation** applies to carbohydrate reactions with proteins **pre-translation**; while **glycation** is reserved for reactions **post-translation**.*

Glycated plasma proteins: fructosamine

HbA_{1c} (see below) is a fructosamine (also known as glycated serum protein (GSP) or glycated albumin); however, in clinical practice the term "**fructosamine**" is usually reserved for **glycated serum proteins**. **Albumin**, the principal protein in plasma, and the other plasma proteins are glycated when exposed to hyperglycaemia, producing fructosamine residues. Since the half-life of albumin is 19 days, the measurement of fructosamine gives an estimation of **average glycaemic control** over the previous **2–3 weeks**.

Haemoglobin A_{1c} (HbA_{1c})

HbA_{1c} (the best-known glycated protein) is a minor component of haemoglobin, formed during the 17-week lifetime of red blood cells when glucose reacts non-enzymatically with the exposed α-amino group of the N-terminal valine of β-globin, forming a fructosamine residue. **The amount of HbA_{1c} formed is determined by the cumulative exposure to the plasma glucose concentration**. Therefore, measurement of HbA_{1c} provides an estimation of the time-averaged glucose concentration during the **8-week period** prior to testing (Table 28.1).

Diabetic ketoacidosis (DKA)

Diabetic ketoacidosis is a complication of diabetes that presents as a medical emergency and is potentially fatal if not treated. Recently in England, during a 12-month period, there were 13,465 emergency admissions for DKA with approximately one-quarter of cases in children and young people under 18 years. DKA is a consequence of complete insulin insufficiency, precipitating a catabolic crisis in which amino acids from muscle protein are converted to glucose (gluconeogenesis; Chapter 34) and fatty acids released from adipose tissue are converted to ketoacids (ketone bodies) (Fig. 33.2), resulting in a significant metabolic acidosis. It has been graphically described as "a melting of the flesh into urine". An exemplary case is shown in Fig. 28.2, where on admission there is severe hyperglycaemia and the **ketone bodies, β-hydroxybutyrate (β-HB)** and **acetoacetate (AcAc)**, are extremely increased with a β-HB:AcAc ratio of 5. Following treatment with insulin, blood glucose and ketone levels decrease, and the β-HB:AcAc ratio falls to a typical value of 3. *NB Urine tests for ketoacidosis usually measure AcAc, which can underestimate its severity.*

Table 28.1 Approximate relationship between the Diabetes Control and Complications Trial (DCCT)-aligned HbA_{1c}, HbA_{1c} and the estimated average glucose concentration based on population studies. This should be used with caution in cases of individual patients. (The reporting of SI units of HbA_{1c} was introduced in 2011.)

DCCT-aligned HbA_{1c} (% of total Hb)	SI units of HbA_{1c} (mmol/mol)	Estimated average glucose	
		mg/dl	mmol/l
4.0	20		
5.0	31		
6.0	42	145	8.1
6.5	48		
7.0	53	180	10.0
7.5	59		
8.0	64	215	11.9
9.0	75	250	13.9
10.0	86	285	15.8
11.0	97	320	17.8
12.0	108	355	19.7

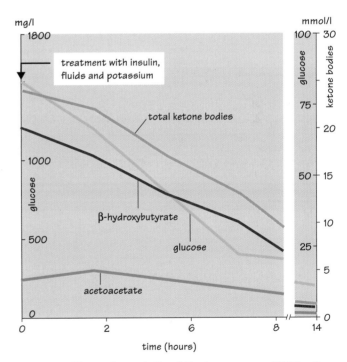

Figure 28.2 Changes in metabolites following treatment of DKA with insulin.

Alcohol metabolism: hypoglycaemia, hyperlactataemia and steatosis

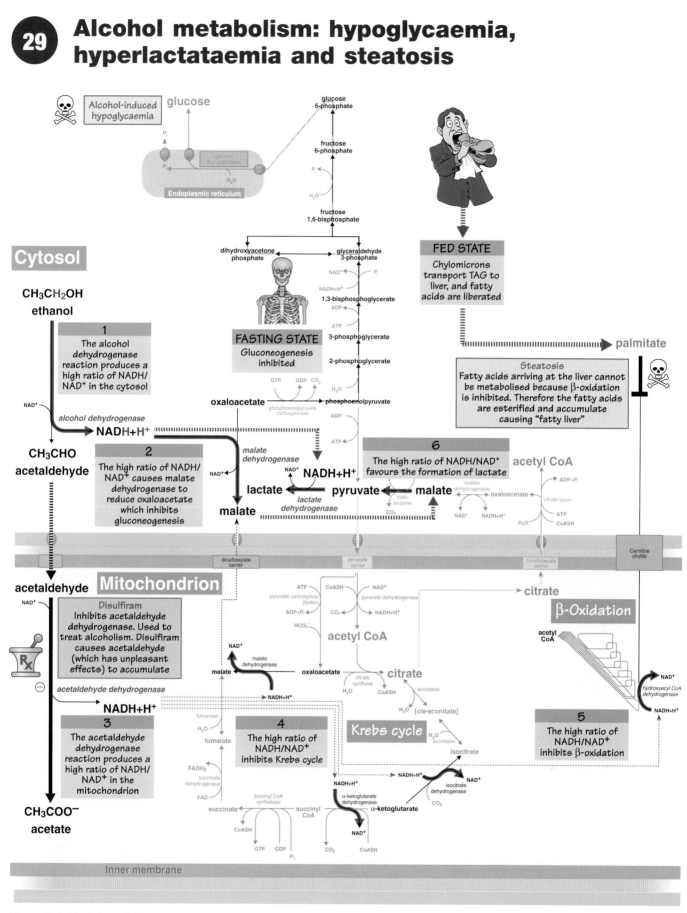

Figure 29.1 Alcohol metabolism.

Ethanol metabolism

Although moderate consumption of ethanol has health benefits, excessive intake causes disease. Ethanol is rapidly metabolised by **alcohol dehydrogenase** in the **cytosol** to form **acetaldehyde**. This requires the coenzyme NAD^+ which is reduced to NADH and results in a **high ratio of $NADH:NAD^+$ in the cytosol**. Subsequently, acetaldehyde is transported into the mitochondrion where it is oxidised by **acetaldehyde dehydrogenase** to **acetate**, which results in a **high mitochondrial ratio of $NADH:NAD^+$**. This elevation of $NADH:NAD^+$ ratios causes the following metabolic consequences of ethanol abuse.

Hypoglycaemia

The high cytosolic ratio of $NADH:NAD^+$ favours reduction of oxaloacetate to malate, redirecting this gluconeogenic precursor away from gluconeogenesis. Anyone who has had a social drink after fasting for a few hours will be familiar with the unpleasant consequences of the fall in blood glucose concentration (remember glucose is the preferred fuel for the brain: a fact which will not be forgotten by my friend Keith*). However, for the habitual alcoholic who regularly neglects food and abuses ethanol the hypoglycaemia can be severe and cause coma.

Hyperlactataemia

Another consequence of the high ratio of cytosolic $NADH:NAD^+$ described above is that lactate dehydrogenase reduces pyruvate to lactate (Fig. 29.1). Moreover, the malate formed as described above is also metabolised to lactate. Therefore ethanol abuse causes hyperlactataemia.

Inhibition of Krebs cycle

Figure 29.1 shows that the high ratio of $NADH:NAD^+$ in the mitochondrion favours reduction of oxaloacetate to malate in the **malate dehydrogenase** reaction. It also restricts oxidation in the α-**ketoglutarate dehydrogenase** and **isocitrate dehydrogenase** reactions. The result is that **Krebs cycle is inhibited**.

Steatosis

Steatosis (fatty liver) is a metabolic consequence of ethanol abuse. This results from a high mitochondrial ratio of $NADH:NAD^+$ which prevents β-oxidation of fatty acids.

Figure 29.1 shows that acetaldehyde is metabolised in liver mitochondria by **acetaldehyde dehydrogenase** to form **acetate**; and NAD^+ forms NADH resulting in a high ratio of $NADH:NAD^+$. This high ratio of $NADH:NAD^+$ prevents oxidation by the **hydroxyacyl CoA dehydrogenase** reaction, therefore β-**oxidation is inhibited**.

Meanwhile, the liver receives fatty acids from dietary lipids. Since these fatty acids cannot be used for β-oxidation, they are esterified and

*By an extraordinary coincidence, while writing this section my friend Keith phoned to say he had just had an accident caused by alcohol-induced hypoglycaemia! He is a busy plant nurseryman and after a hectic day (minimal breakfast, skipped lunch, much physical exercise, no evening meal; all contriving to exhaust his liver glycogen reserves) he rushed to sing in an evening performance with his choral society. He had a convivial glass of wine before the show. During the programme he began to sweat, felt dizzy and fell, not alas forwards into the warm embrace of the sopranos, but backwards off the podium. He awoke on the way to hospital with a fractured fibula!

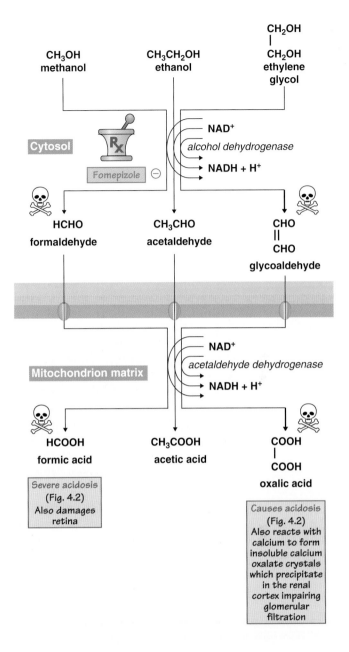

Figure 29.2 Metabolism of methanol and ethylene glycol.

accumulate in the liver as triacylglycerol (TAG), a condition known as steatosis.

Methanol and ethylene glycol form toxic products

Methanol is used as antifreeze and is also added to ethanol as a denaturant. Similarly, ethylene glycol is used as an antifreeze, especially in automobiles. Both compounds themselves are not toxic, but following ingestion they are metabolised rapidly by alcohol dehydrogenase to metabolites (**formic acid** and **oxalic acid**) which are potentially lethal. **Fomepizole** (4-methylpyrazone) **inhibits alcohol dehydrogenase** and is used clinically to treat methanol and ethylene glycol toxicity.

30 Enzymes: nomenclature, kinetics and inhibitors

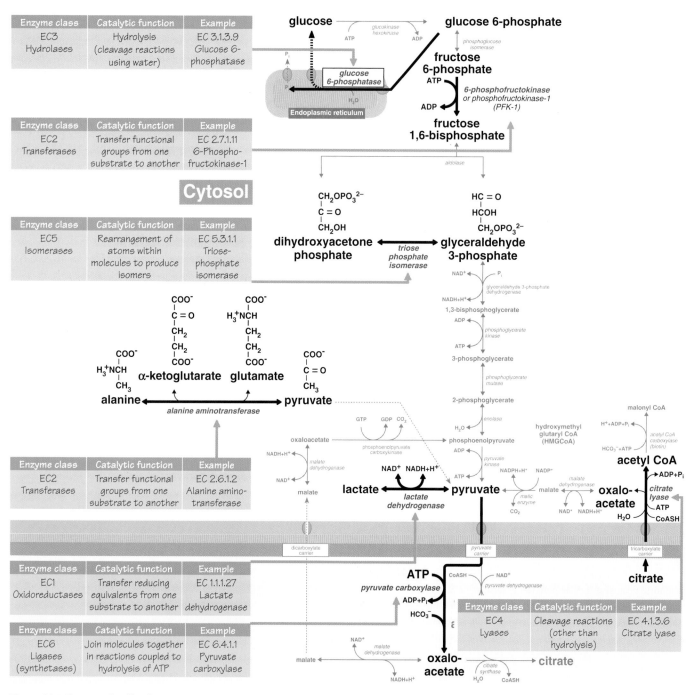

Figure 30.1 Enzyme classification.

Enzyme nomenclature

Enzyme nomenclature and classification is according to recommendations of the International Union of Biochemistry and Molecular Biology (**IUBMB**) www.chem.qmul.ac.uk/iubmb. Enzymes are classified in **six classes** (**EC1**, **EC2**, **EC3**, etc.), which in turn are divided into subclasses (Fig. 30.1).

Enzyme kinetics: velocity versus substrate concentration curve

Figure 30.2 shows an initial velocity versus substrate concentration curve. The reaction velocity (v) increases in proportion to increasing concentration of substrate [S] until all the catalytic sites of the enzyme are working as fast as they can and maximum reaction velocity (V_{max})

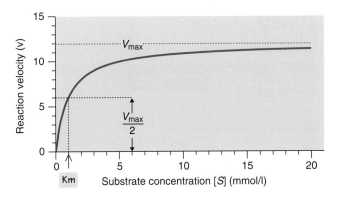

Figure 30.2 Michaelis–Menten plot.

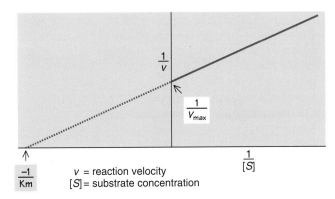

Figure 30.3 Lineweaver–Burke double reciprocal plot.

v = reaction velocity
$[S]$ = substrate concentration

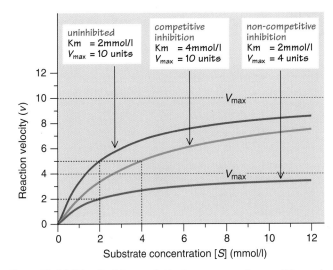

Figure 30.4 Michaelis–Menten plot in the presence of competitive and non-competitive inhibitors.

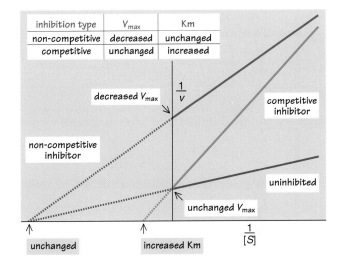

Figure 30.5 Lineweaver–Burke double reciprocal plot in the presence of competitive and non-competitive inhibitors.

Competitive and non-competitive inhibition

Figure 30.4 shows the Michaelis–Menten v versus $[S]$ plot for an enzyme in the absence and presence of either competitive or non-competitive inhibitors. Figure 30.5 shows the same as a Lineweaver–Burke reciprocal plot. Figure 30.4 also shows an uninhibited enzyme that has a V_{max} of 10 units and a Km of 2 mmol/l.

Competitive enzyme inhibitors are used as drugs. They have structures similar to the natural substrate and can therefore compete with it for access to the same binding site on the enzyme. For example, **methotrexate** (an anticancer drug) structurally resembles **folate**, which is the natural substrate for **dihydrofolate reductase** (Chapter 58). Methotrexate is used to inhibit dihydrofolate reductase in cancer chemotherapy.

In Fig. 30.4 we see how an enzyme in the presence of a competitor needs more substrate to beat off the competition. However, given sufficient substrate the competitive inhibitor is overwhelmed, inhibition

(12 units) is approached. From this graph the Michaelis–Menten constant (Km) is obtained. The Km is defined as "the substrate concentration giving half V_{max} ($V_{max}/2$)". In Fig. 30.2 the Km is 1 mmol/l.

If the substrate concentration and reaction velocity are plotted as the reciprocal of their values, a linear relationship known as the Lineweaver–Burke plot is obtained (Fig. 30.3).

is reversed, and the enzyme can operate at its normal V_{max}. NB The competitor obstructs the binding site thus **decreasing** the affinity of the enzyme for its substrate, in other words it **increases** the Km, e.g. to 4 mmol/l but V_{max} is unchanged.

Non-competitive inhibitors bind to sites other than the substrate binding site, therefore inhibition is not overcome by increasing the substrate concentration. In fact, non-competitive inhibition is simply understood by remembering that each substrate has its own sub-binding site. Therefore, increasing the concentration of one substrate will not alter the binding of an inhibitor that is blocking another sub-binding site. Consequently, non-competitive inhibitors affect a fixed proportion of the enzyme molecules, do not change the Km, but decrease V_{max} by a constant percentage.

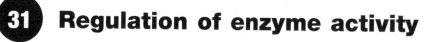

31 Regulation of enzyme activity

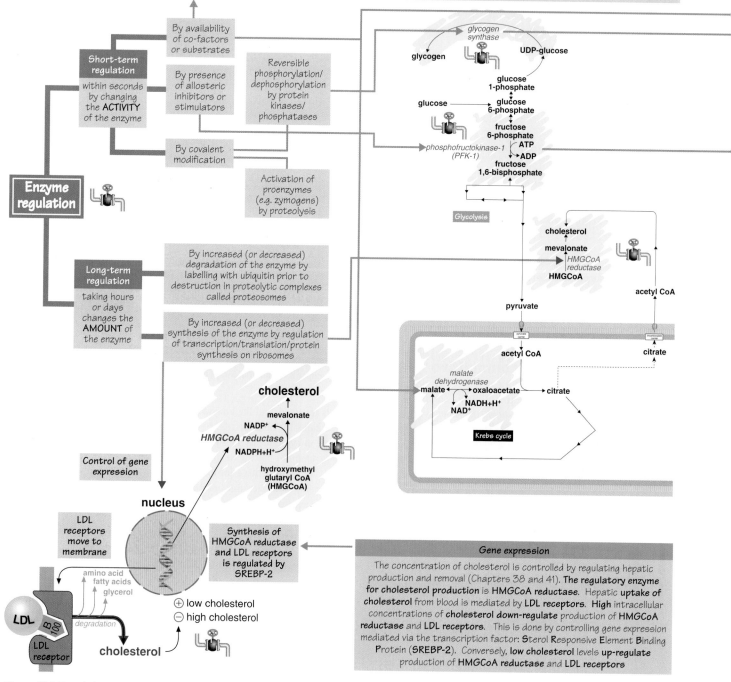

Figure 31.1 Regulation of enzyme activity.

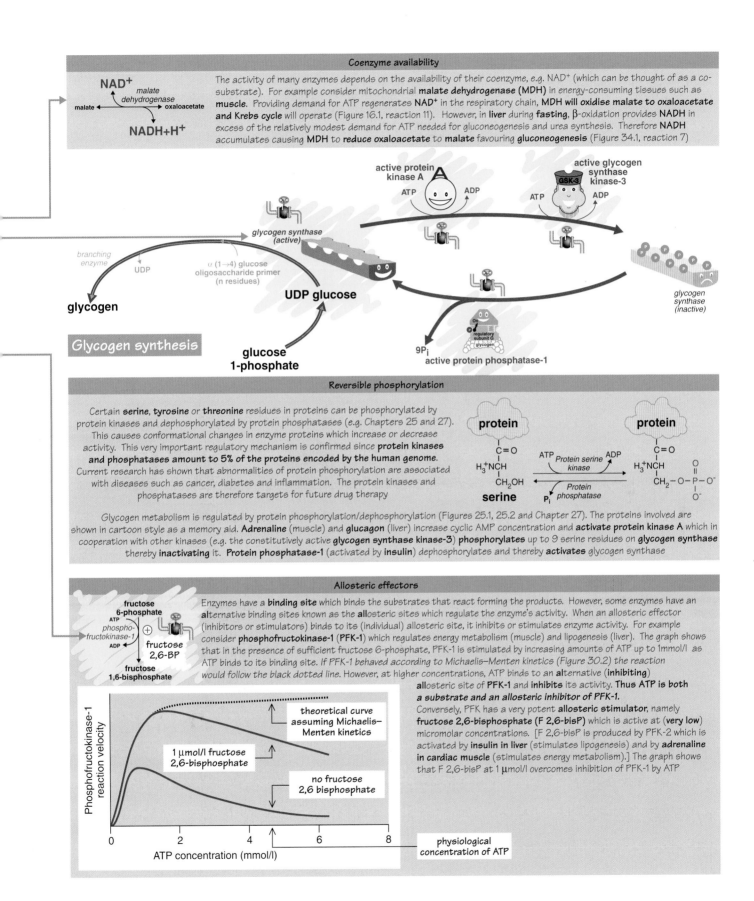

The activity of many enzymes depends on the availability of their coenzyme, e.g. NAD⁺ (which can be thought of as a co-substrate). For example consider mitochondrial **malate dehydrogenase (MDH)** in energy-consuming tissues such as **muscle**. Providing demand for ATP regenerates **NAD⁺** in the respiratory chain, MDH will oxidise malate to oxaloacetate and **Krebs cycle** will operate (Figure 16.1, reaction 11). However, in **liver** during **fasting**, β-oxidation provides NADH in excess of the relatively modest demand for ATP needed for gluconeogenesis and urea synthesis. Therefore NADH accumulates causing **MDH** to **reduce oxaloacetate** to **malate** favouring **gluconeogenesis** (Figure 34.1, reaction 7)

Glycogen synthesis

Reversible phosphorylation

Certain **serine, tyrosine** or **threonine** residues in proteins can be phosphorylated by protein kinases and dephosphorylated by protein phosphatases (e.g. Chapters 25 and 27). This causes conformational changes in enzyme proteins which increase or decrease activity. This very important regulatory mechanism is confirmed since **protein kinases and phosphatases amount to 5% of the proteins encoded by the human genome.** Current research has shown that abnormalities of protein phosphorylation are associated with diseases such as cancer, diabetes and inflammation. The protein kinases and phosphatases are therefore targets for future drug therapy

Glycogen metabolism is regulated by protein phosphorylation/dephosphorylation (Figures 25.1, 25.2 and Chapter 27). The proteins involved are shown in cartoon style as a memory aid. **Adrenaline** (muscle) and **glucagon** (liver) increase cyclic AMP concentration and **activate protein kinase A** which in cooperation with other kinases (e.g. the constitutively active **glycogen synthase kinase-3**) **phosphorylates** up to 9 serine residues on **glycogen synthase** thereby **inactivating** it. **Protein phosphatase-1** (activated by **insulin**) dephosphorylates and thereby **activates** glycogen synthase

Allosteric effectors

Enzymes have a **binding site** which binds the substrates that react forming the products. However, some enzymes have an **alternative binding sites** known as the **allosteric sites** which regulate the enzyme's activity. When an allosteric effector (inhibitors or stimulators) binds to its (individual) allosteric site, it inhibits or stimulates enzyme activity. For example consider **phosphofructokinase-1** (PFK-1) which regulates energy metabolism (muscle) and lipogenesis (liver). The graph shows that in the presence of sufficient fructose 6-phosphate, PFK-1 is stimulated by increasing amounts of ATP up to 1mmol/l as ATP binds to its binding site. If PFK-1 behaved according to Michaelis–Menten kinetics (Figure 30.2) the reaction would follow the black dotted line. However, at higher concentrations, ATP binds to an alternative (inhibiting) allosteric site of PFK-1 and **inhibits** its activity. **Thus ATP is both a substrate and an allosteric inhibitor of PFK-1.**

Conversely, PFK has a very potent **allosteric stimulator**, namely **fructose 2,6-bisphosphate (F 2,6-bisP)** which is active at (**very low**) micromolar concentrations. [F 2,6-bisP is produced by PFK-2 which is activated by **insulin in liver** (stimulates lipogenesis) and by **adrenaline in cardiac muscle** (stimulates energy metabolism).] The graph shows that F 2,6-bisP at 1 μmol/l overcomes inhibition of PFK-1 by ATP

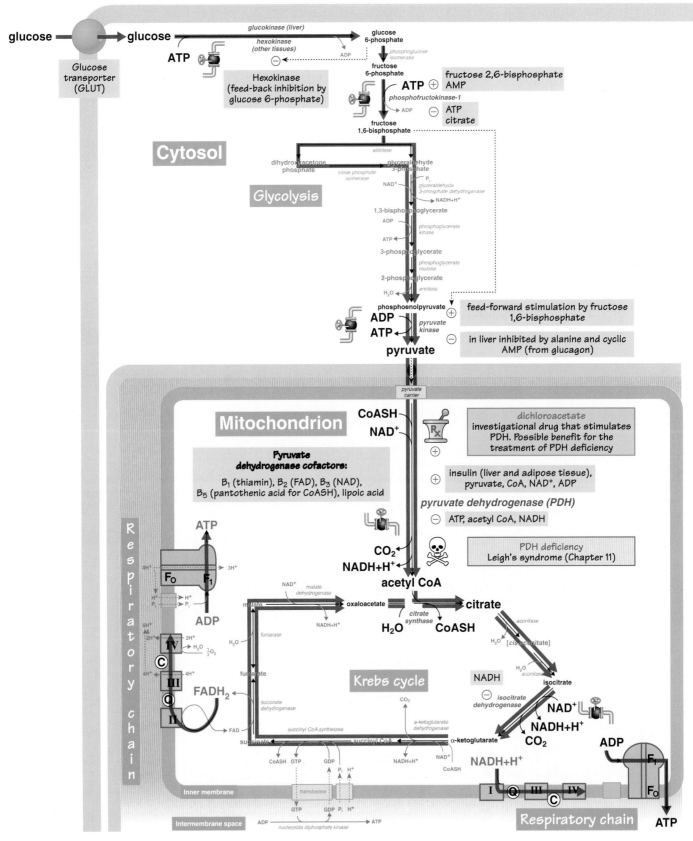

Figure 32.1 Regulation of glycolysis and Krebs cycle.

Regulation of glycolysis

Glycolysis has different functions in different tissues. In **anaerobic** tissues such as white muscle, retina and in red blood cells, its main function is the production of ATP with lactate as the end product (Chapter 17). Under **aerobic** conditions in muscle, glycolysis provides pyruvate for oxidation in Krebs cycle which cooperates with the respiratory chain to make ATP. In liver and adipose tissue, glycolysis co-operates with the pentose phosphate pathway to produce pyruvate for fatty acid synthesis (Fig. 21.2). *NB Nature has good reasons for its design of metabolic regulation! When studying metabolic pathways, remember that the regulation of metabolism is directed to their functions.*

Glycolysis is regulated by: (i) **glucose transporters (GLUTs)**, (ii) **glucokinase** or **hexokinase**, (iii) **phosphofructokinase 1**, (iv) **pyruvate kinase**, and (v) **pyruvate dehydrogenase**.

Glucose transporters (GLUTs)

Glucose enters a cell via **glucose transporters (GLUTs)**. There are several types, e.g. **GLUT1**, **GLUT2**, etc. Glucose transporters are located in the plasma membrane, except for **GLUT4**, which controls glycolysis in **muscle** and **adipose tissue**. During fasting, **GLUT4** transporters are located in intracellular vesicles. After feeding, **insulin** causes the vesicles to recruit GLUT4 into the plasma membrane enabling glucose transport into the cell (Fig. 27.1).

Glucokinase and hexokinase

The first reaction of glycolysis is the phosphorylation of glucose to glucose 6-phosphate, catalysed by hexokinase or glucokinase. **Hexokinase** is found in most types of cell and has a low Km (i.e. a high affinity) for glucose, and is subject to feed-back inhibition by **glucose 6-phosphate**. Glucokinase has a high Km (i.e. low affinity) for glucose and is found in liver and the β-cells of pancreas. In liver, it is well adapted to cope with the high concentrations of glucose (up to 15 mmol/l) transported from the intestines by the hepatic portal vein after a carbohydrate meal. *Remember: gLucokinase is found in the Liver.*

Phosphofructokinase 1 (PFK-1)

Stimulation of PFK-1: **PFK-1** is stimulated by **fructose 2,6-bisphosphate (F 2,6-bisP)**. PFK-1 is also stimulated by **AMP** which, when abundant, indicates a **low** energy state and the need for ATP synthesis requiring increased glycolysis.

*NB Production of F 2,6-bisP is **stimulated** by insulin in liver, and by high fructose 6-phosphate concentrations in skeletal muscle. F 2,6-bisP is **depleted** by glucagon in liver, and by low fructose 6-phosphate concentrations in skeletal muscle.*

Inhibition of PFK-1: When **ATP** is abundant, it inhibits PFK-1 and restricts glycolysis. Another inhibitor of PFK-1 is **citrate**.

Pyruvate kinase (PK)

Inhibition of PK In **liver**, pyruvate kinase is **inhibited** by **alanine** and **cyclic AMP** (which is produced under the influence of **glucagon**). Glucagon is present during fasting, as is the gluconeogenic precursor alanine, which is derived from muscle protein (Chapter 44). Inhibition of PK restricts phosphoenolpyruvate catabolism and favours gluconeogenesis (Fig. 46.2).

Stimulation of PK In **liver**, pyruvate kinase is **stimulated** by **fructose 1,6-bisphosphate** (feed-forward stimulation). This is especially important during the transition from fasting (gluconeogenesis, PK inhibited) to lipogenesis (PK active) (Chapter 21).

Pyruvate dehydrogenase (PDH)

PDH is a complex of three enzymes located in the mitochondrion. It controls the rate of entry of pyruvate into Krebs cycle.

Stimulation of PDH After a carbohydrate meal, PDH is **stimulated** by **insulin** in liver and adipose tissue where pyruvate is destined for fatty acid synthesis (Chapter 21). PDH is also stimulated by its substrate **pyruvate**, and by the availability of its coenzymes **CoA** and **NAD$^+$**. Finally, PDH is stimulated by **ADP**, which is increased in the low energy state and indicates the need for ATP synthesis by co-operation of Krebs cycle and the respiratory chain.

Inhibition of PDH PDH is inhibited by **ATP** when it is abundant, thereby restricting the oxidation of pyruvate by Krebs cycle. PDH is also inhibited by **acetyl CoA** and **NADH**, which are products of the PDH reaction. When acetyl CoA and NADH are abundant, fatty acids are used as metabolic fuel and their inhibition of pyruvate dehydrogenase helps to conserves pyruvate (NB during starvation, pyruvate is made from food reserves, e.g. glycogen and amino acids derived from muscle protein (Chapter 46)).

Regulation of Krebs cycle

Krebs cycle has different functions in different tissues. For example, in **muscle** and **brain** it oxidises acetyl CoA to form NADH and FADH$_2$, which are used to generate ATP in the respiratory chain (Chapters 11–13). In **liver**, **during fasting**, acetyl CoA is not oxidised by Krebs cycle. Instead, sections of Krebs cycle operate to direct amino acid derivatives towards malate for gluconeogenesis (Chapter 46). In **liver** and **adipose tissue**, **after feeding**, the destiny of acetyl CoA is a brief sojourn in Krebs cycle by incorporation into citrate before export to the cytosol for biosynthesis to fatty acids (Chapter 21).

Isocitrate dehydrogenase (ICDH)

ICDH is inhibited when NADH accumulates. This is obvious when it is realised that the coenzyme for ICDH is NAD$^+$, which is depleted when it has been reduced to NADH.

Disorders of PDH activity
Thiamin deficiency

Nerve tissue is mainly dependent for ATP production on glucose metabolism via glycolysis to produce acetyl CoA by the PDH reaction for oxidation in Krebs cycle. Since thiamin is essential for PDH activity, thiamin deficiency, which can occur in malnourished alcoholics, results in PDH dysfunction and an energy deficit in nerve tissue. This causes hyperlactataemia and neuropathy, which can progress to Wernicke's encephalopathy and Korsakoff's psychosis (Chapter 53).

Remember that although fatty acids produce acetyl CoA independently of PDH, they are not available to the brain for fuel as they cannot cross the blood–brain barrier.

Leigh's syndrome

Some forms of Leigh's syndrome are caused by PDH dysfunction (Chapter 11).

Yield of ATP from the complete oxidation of palmitate		
Reaction	**NADH or FADH$_2$**	**ATP yield**
1 Long-chain acyl CoA synthetase		−2
2 Acyl CoA dehydrogenase (× 7)	7 FADH$_2$	10.5
3 L-3-hydroxyacyl CoA dehydrogenase (× 7)	7 NADH	17.5
4 Isocitrate dehydrogenase	8 NADH	20
5 α-Ketoglutarate dehydrogenase	8 NADH	20
6 Succinyl CoA synthetase/nucleoside diphosphate kinase		8
7 Succinate dehydrogenase	8 FADH$_2$	12
8 Malate dehydrogenase	8 NADH	20
	TOTAL	106

NB The total of 106 does not allow for the energy used to transport phosphate (equivalent to 2 ATPs) so true net yield is 104 ATP, see JG Salway, *Metabolism at a Glance*, 3rd ed pp 38–9, Blackwell Publishing

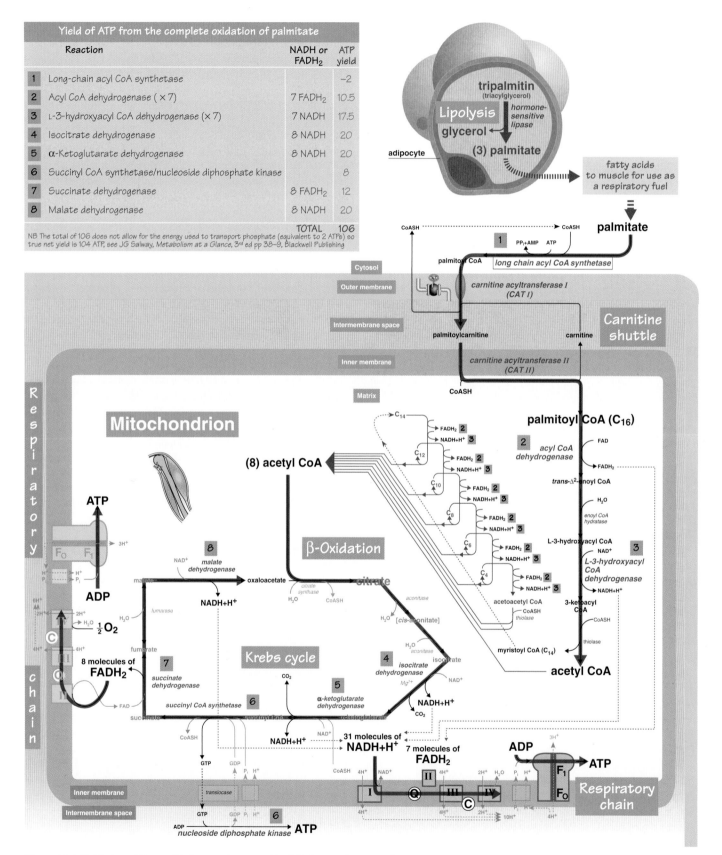

Figure 33.1 Oxidation of fatty acids by muscle to provide ATP for muscle contraction.

Medical Biochemistry at a Glance, Third Edition. J. G. Salway. © 2012 John Wiley & Sons, Ltd. Published 2012 by John Wiley & Sons, Ltd.

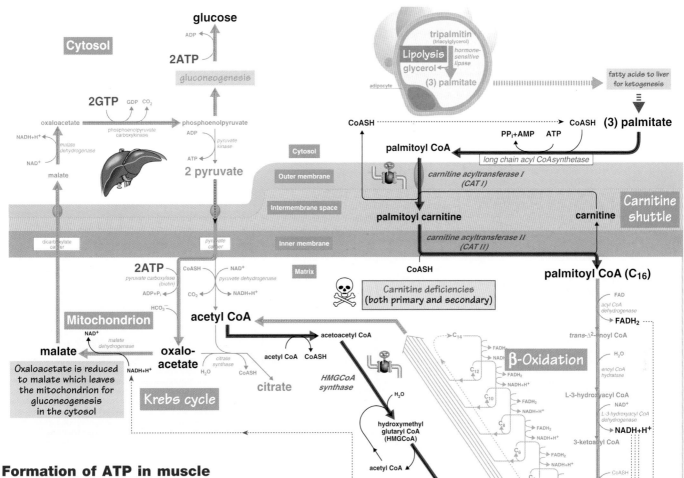

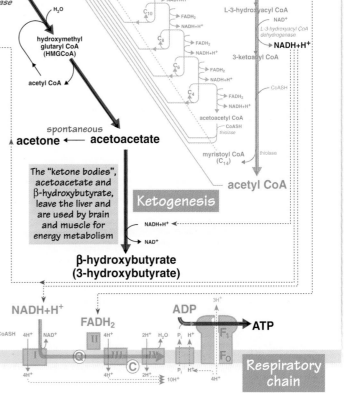

Formation of ATP in muscle

Under aerobic conditions, fatty acids are the fuel preferred by muscle and undergo β-oxidation to produce ATP (Fig. 33.1).

Formation of ATP and ketone bodies in liver

During fasting or in uncontrolled diabetes mellitus, fatty acids enter liver cells and are transported from the cytosol into the mitochondrion (Fig. 33.2). *NB The **carnitine shuttle** is needed to transport fatty acids into the mitochondrial matrix.*

Carnitine shuttle

Palmitoyl CoA combines with **carnitine** in a reaction catalysed by **carnitine acyltransferase I** (**CAT I**) located in the mitochondrial **outer** membrane, to form **palmitoyl carnitine**. The palmitoyl CoA is regenerated from **palmitoyl carnitine** by **carnitine acyltransferase II** (**CAT II**) located in the mitochondrial **inner** membrane.

In carnitine deficiency, fatty acids cannot enter the mitochondrion. Consequently β-oxidation is inhibited, resulting in hypoglycaemia.

Ketogenesis

Fatty acids undergo β-oxidation, producing acetyl CoA, NADH and $FADH_2$. The NADH and $FADH_2$ are oxidised by the respiratory chain to form ATP which is used for gluconeogenesis (Chapter 34) and for urea synthesis (Chapter 44). The acetyl CoA forms the ketoacids **acetoacetate** and **β-hydroxybutyrate**, known as the "**ketone bodies**". **Acetone**, formed in small amounts from acetoacetate, causes the fruity smell of the breath in ketotic patients or people on low carbohydrate diets (e.g. the "Atkins diet"). NB When the ratio of $NADH:NAD^+$ is high, as in **diabetic ketoacidosis** (**DKA**), the equilibrium of the β-

Figure 33.2 Oxidation of fatty acids by liver to provide ATP for gluconeogenesis and acetyl CoA for ketogenesis.

hydroxybutyrate dehydrogenase reaction favours β-hydroxybutyrate production (Fig. 28.2). Hence acetoacetate in DKA can be 20% of the β-hydroxybutyrate concentration. **Warning**: the nitroprusside reaction used to detect "ketone bodies" in urine measures only acetoacetate and **not** the principal ketone body, β-hydroxybutyrate.

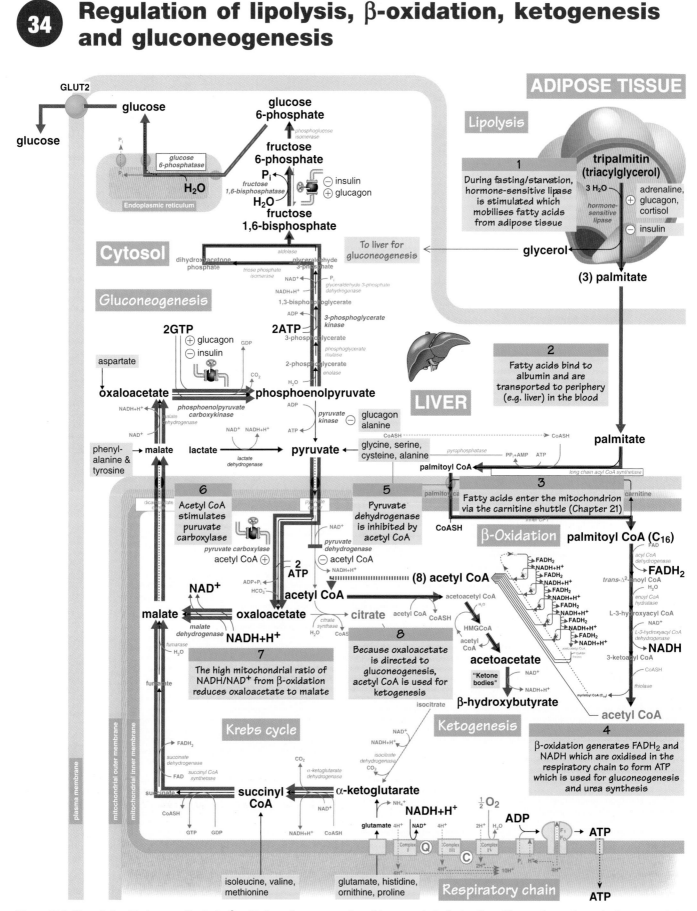

Figure 34.1 The relationship between lipolysis, β-oxidation, gluconeogenesis and ketogenesis in fasting liver (the numbers refer to the box, *opposite*).

The liver maintains blood glucose during starvation

The principal fuel for the brain is glucose. If brain is deprived of glucose (**neuroglycopenia**) the result is coma. Patients with **insulinoma** produce excessive amounts of insulin resulting in hypoglycaemia, fainting or abnormal behaviour which can be misdiagnosed as epilepsy or psychiatric illness. Similarly, patients with type 1 diabetes are familiar with the symptoms of hypoglycaemia and the need to prevent a "hypo" by balancing their food intake with their insulin injections.

The normal fasting blood glucose concentration is maintained between 3.5 and 5.5 mmol/l. This remarkable feat of metabolic control applies despite extremes of metabolic stress; for example, during the sudden huge demand for fuel by a 100-metre sprinter (glucose from muscle glycogen) or the longer term, massive fuel consumption needed by a Marathon runner (fatty acids from adipose tissue plus glucose from both muscle and liver glycogen). Moreover, blood glucose must be maintained above 3.5 mmol/l during short-term fasting or long-term starvation over several weeks. The liver plays a vital role in glucose homeostasis (Chapter 23).

Liver glycogen

During the first few hours of fasting, **glucagon** activates glycogen breakdown in the liver (glycogenolysis), which releases glucose into the blood, preventing hypoglycaemia (Fig. 26.1).

Fuels used when liver glycogen is exhausted
Gluconeogenesis

Liver glycogen is exhausted within 24 hours. **NB THE BRAIN CANNOT USE FATTY ACIDS AS A FUEL and FATTY ACIDS CANNOT BE METABOLISED TO GLUCOSE.** So, within 24 hours, the carbohydrate reserve (i.e. glycogen) is exhausted. Since fatty acids from triacylglycerol cannot be used as fuel by the brain, the principal remaining brain fuel is glucose, which is made from muscle protein. Desperate needs demand desperate measures! So within 24 hours of starvation, the glucocorticoid hormone cortisol directs the metabolic pathways to break down muscle (muscle-wasting!) to form amino acids, some of which can be metabolised to glucose by **gluconeogenesis. NB This emphasises the importance of nutrition in patients recovering from tissue trauma whether surgical, burns or crush injury. Wound healing will be slow if the patient does not eat and is in a gluconeogenic (muscle-wasting) catabolic state.**

Ketogenesis

The liver makes ketone bodies from fatty acids during fasting. Fortunately, after 2 days of fasting, the brain adapts to use the ketone bodies as fuel, reducing the need for glucose and therefore decreasing the need for gluconeogenesis.

Regulation of lipolysis

Lipolysis is the process by which **fatty acids** and **glycerol** are mobilised from the triacylglycerol reserves in **white adipose tissue**. The regulatory enzyme of lipolysis is **hormone-sensitive lipase**, which is stimulated by the hormones secreted during fasting, namely **glucagon** and **cortisol**. In the fed state, **insulin** inhibits hormone-sensitive lipase thus favouring triacylglycerol accumulation. *NB Lipolysis produces glycerol, which is a gluconeogenic substrate and is metabolised to glucose.*

The fatty acids released from adipose tissue are insoluble in the aqueous environment of the blood and bind to albumin, which transports them in the blood to the periphery.

Regulation of β-oxidation

The fatty acids must be transported into the mitochondrion where β-oxidation occurs. Transport of fatty acids through the inner mitochondrial membrane involves the **carnitine shuttle** (Chapter 21). The carnitine shuttle is inhibited by **malonyl CoA** which inactivates **carnitine acyltransferase I (CAT I)**. Malonyl CoA is produced when fatty acids are being synthesised during the fed state, and by inhibiting the carnitine shuttle it prevents the futile destruction by β-oxidation of the brand-new fatty acids as they are formed.

Regulation of gluconeogenesis

The regulatory enzymes of gluconeogenesis are confined to the liver and kidney.

1 Pyruvate carboxylase in the mitochondrion needs ATP and biotin, is induced by cortisol and is stimulated by acetyl CoA.

2 Phosphoenolpyruvate carboxykinase (PEPCK) in the cytosol needs GTP, is stimulated by glucagon and inhibited by insulin.

3 Fructose 1,6-bisphosphatase (F 1,6-bisPase) in the cytosol is inhibited by **fructose 2,6-bisphosphate**. Fructose 2,6-bisphosphate is destroyed under the influence of glucagon. Conversely, it is synthesised under the influence of insulin.

4 Glucose 6-phosphatase is in the endoplasmic reticulum.

Regulation of ketogenesis

The rate of ketogenesis increases in proportion to the blood fatty acid concentration. It increases during fasting and especially in uncontrolled type 1 diabetes (**diabetic ketoacidosis (DKA)**).

---

1 During fasting or starvation, the catabolic hormones **glucagon** and **cortisol** are secreted from the α-cells of the pancreas and the adrenal cortex, respectively. In response to severe stress or danger, adrenaline is secreted by the adrenal medulla. **These hormones stimulate hormone-sensitive lipase that mobilises fatty acids and glycerol from white adipose tissue.**

2 The **fatty acids** bind to albumin and are transported in the blood to the liver.

3 Fatty acids enter the mitochondrion via the carnitine shuttle.

4 β-Oxidation of the fatty acids generates $FADH_2$ and NADH and acetyl CoA. $FADH_2$ and NADH are oxidised in the respiratory chain to supply ATP for gluconeogenesis.

5 Acetyl CoA inhibits pyruvate dehydrogenase.

6 Acetyl CoA stimulates pyruvate carboxylase, which converts pyruvate to oxaloacetate.

7 β-Oxidation ensures that the mitochondrial ratio $NADH:NAD^+$ is high. The high proportion of NADH reduces **oxaloacetate** to **malate**. Malate is transported from the mitochondrion into the cytosol where it forms glucose by the process of **gluconeogenesis**.

8 Gluconeogenesis is the production of glucose from non-carbohydrate substrates, e.g. amino acids. NB 6 ATP equivalents (from β-oxidation, see (4)) are needed to produce 1 glucose molecule.

Ketogenesis: mitochondrial oxaloacetate is depleted. Therefore, acetyl CoA cannot react with oxaloacetate to form citrate for oxidation in Krebs cycle. Instead, acetyl CoA reacts with itself to form **acetoacetate and 3-hydroxybutyrate (the ketone bodies).**

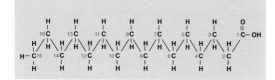

Figure 35.1 Glycerol. A carbohydrate that forms the "backbone" of triacylglycerols (TAGs).

Figure 35.2 Palmitic acid (hexadecanoic acid). A C_{16} saturated fatty acid, i.e. it has 16 carbon atoms, all of which (apart from the C1 carboxylic acid group) are **fully saturated** with hydrogen.

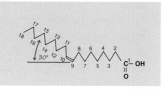

Figure 35.3 Stearic acid (octadecanoic acid). A C_{18} saturated fatty acid, i.e. it has 18 carbon atoms, all of which (apart from the C1 carboxylic acid group) are **fully saturated** with hydrogen. This simplified representation of the structure does not show the hydrogen atoms.

Figure 35.4 *cis*-Oleic acid. A $C_{18:1}$ **mono**-unsaturated fatty acid, i.e. it has **one** double bond at C9, and so the carbon atoms C9 and C10 are not saturated with their full capacity of two hydrogen atoms each. NB The double bond creates a 30° angle. (*cis*- and *trans*- are defined in Fig. 35.14.)

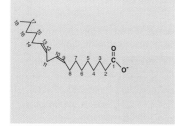

Figure 35.5 Linoleic acid. A $C_{18:2}$ poly-unsaturated fatty acid, i.e. it has 18 carbon atoms and **two** ***cis*-unsaturated bonds** at C9 and C12.

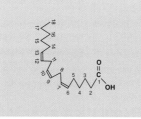

Figure 35.6 γ-Linolenic acid. A $C_{18:3}$ poly-unsaturated fatty acid, i.e. it has 18 carbon atoms and **three** ***cis*-unsaturated bonds** at C6, C9 and C12.

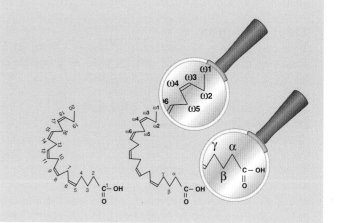

Figure 35.8 Eicosapentaenoic acid (EPA). A $C_{20:5}$ poly-unsaturated fatty acid, i.e. it has 20 carbon atoms and **five *cis*-unsaturated bonds** at C5, C8, C11, C14 and C17. **Nomenclature:** NB There is an alternative system for identifying the carbon atoms of fatty acids which is popular with nutritionists and uses Greek letters. The carboxylic acid group is ignored and the next carbon is α-, then β-, γ-, etc. until the last carbon which is the last letter of the Greek alphabet, ω-. The system then counts backwards from ω, so we have ω1, ω2, ω3, etc. Thus EPA, which is an essential fatty acid found in fish oil, is classified as a ω3 fatty acid. *(Chemists (who claim to be the prima donnas of chemical nomenclature) prefer to label the last carbon "n", so chemists refer to **n1, n2, n3**, etc.)*

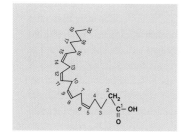

Figure 35.7 Arachidonic acid. A $C_{20:4}$ poly-unsaturated fatty acid, i.e. it has 20 carbon atoms and **four** ***cis*-unsaturated bonds** at C5, C8, C11 and C14. NB Arachidonic acid is sometimes mispronounced "arach-**nid**-onic". Note that it is derived from peanuts (ground nuts; Greek *arakos*) and *not* from spiders (arachnids)!

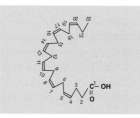

Figure 35.9 Docosahexaenoic acid (DHA). A $C_{22:6}$ poly-unsaturated fatty acid, i.e. it has 22 carbon atoms and **six *cis*-unsaturated bonds** at C4, C7, C10, C13, C16 and C20. DHA is an essential fatty acid found in fish oil, and is a ω3 fatty acid.

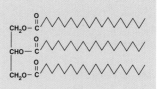

Figure 35.10 Triacylglycerol (TAG or triglyceride). TAG consists of **three** fatty **acyl** groups esterified with a **glycerol** backbone, hence the name **triacylglycerol**. The fatty acids can vary, but in the example shown all three are **stearic** acid so this TAG is called "**tristearin**". *(In clinical circles the term "**triglyceride**" is commonly used. This incorrectly suggests that the molecule comprises "three glycerols" and so has been rejected by chemists.)*

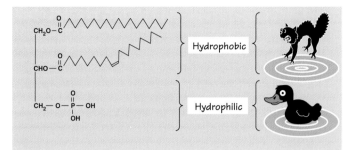

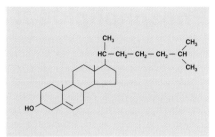

Figure 35.12 Cholesterol.

Figure 35.11 **Phosphatidic acid**. This is the "parent" molecule of the phospholipids. Like triacylglycerol, it has a glycerol backbone but instead comprises two fatty acyl groups and one phosphate group. When this phosphate reacts with OH groups of compounds such as choline, ethanolamine, serine or inositol, phospholipids are formed known as **phosphatidylcholine, phosphatidylethanolamine, phosphatidylserine** and **phosphatidylinositol** (Chapter 36).

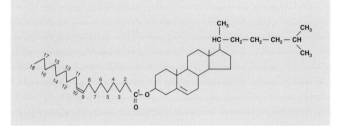

Figure 35.13 **Cholesteryl ester**. When cholesterol is esterified with a fatty acid, cholesteryl ester is formed.

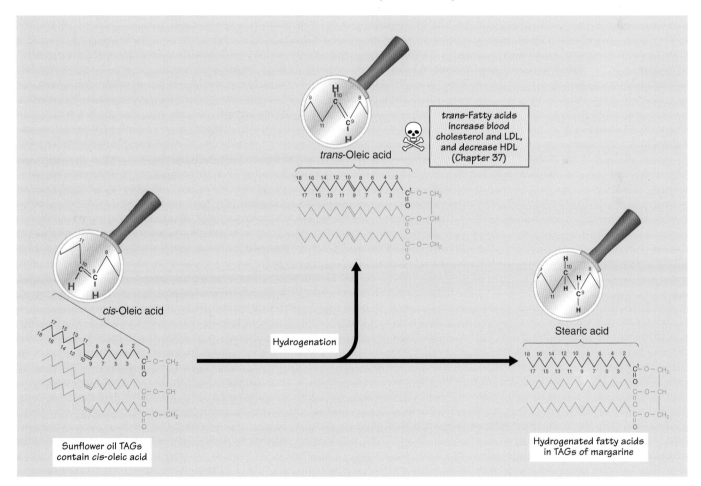

Figure 35.14 *cis*- and *trans*-**fatty acids**. The terms *cis*- and *trans*- refer to the position of molecules around a double bond. In *cis*-oleic acid, the hydrogen atoms are on the **same side** of the double bond, whereas in *trans*-oleic acid, the hydrogen atoms are on **opposite sides** of the double bond. (Think of transatlantic, opposite sides of the Atlantic Ocean.) Notice that *trans*-fatty acids do not have the 30° angle in their chain. The result is that, although they are unsaturated, they are both structurally and physiologically more like saturated fatty acids. Unfortunately, *trans*-fatty acids can be formed in the hydrogenation process during margarine manufacture which converts the fatty acyl groups of TAG in sunflower oil (a fluid) to (solid) margarine. Nowadays, many countries ban *trans*-fatty acids from food products.

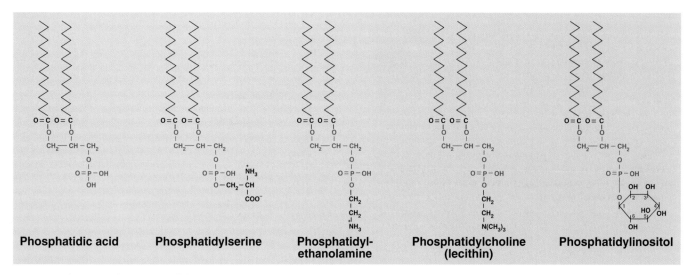

Figure 36.1 Structure of the phospholipids.

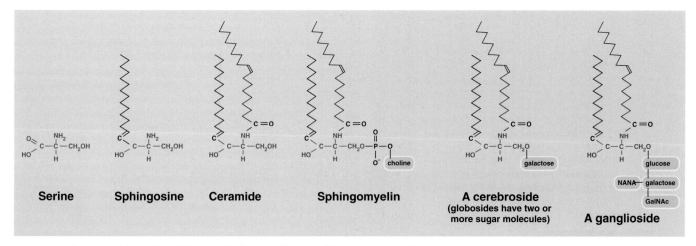

Figure 36.2 Structure of the sphingolipids. NB Sphingomyelin is classified as a phospholipid.

Phospholipids

Phospholipids are important components of cell membranes and lipoproteins (Chapter 37). They are **amphipathic** compounds, i.e. they have an affinity for both aqueous and non-aqueous environments. The **hydrophobic** part of the molecule associates with **hydrophobic lipid molecules**, while the **hydrophilic** part of the molecule associates with **water**. In this way, phospholipids are compounds that form bridges between water and lipids.

The parent molecule of the phospholipid family is **phosphatidic acid** (Fig. 36.1). It consists of a **glycerol** "backbone" to which are esterified **two fatty acyl molecules** (palmitic acid is shown here) and phosphoric acid. The latter produces a **phosphate** which is free to react with the hydroxyl groups of **serine, ethanolamine, choline** or **inositol** to form **phosphatidylserine, phosphatidylethanolamine, phosphatidylcholine** or **phosphatidylinositol**, respectively.

Phosphatidylcholine

This is also known as **lecithin** and is frequently used in food as an emulsifying agent whereby it causes lipids to associate with water molecules.

Respiratory distress syndrome

Respiratory distress syndrome (RDS) is a common problem in premature infants. The immature lung fails to produce dipalmitoyllecithin, which is a surfactant. RDS occurs when the alveoli collapse inwards after expiration and adhere under the prevailing surface tension (atelectasis). The function of dipalmitoyllecithin is to reduce the surface tension and permit expansion of the alveoli on inflation. Assessment of the maturity of foetal lung function can be made by measuring the ratio of **lecithin** to **sphingomyelin** (the **L/S ratio**) in amniotic fluid.

Phosphatidylinositol

This is the parent molecule of the phosphoinositides, e.g. **phosphatidylinositol 3,4,5-trisphosphate** (**PIP_3**) which is involved in insulin-stimulated intracellular signal transduction (Chapter 27).

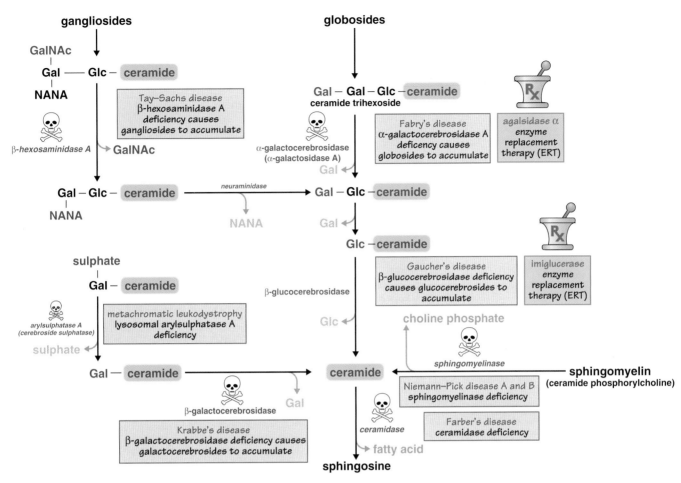

Figure 36.3 Degradation of the sphingolipids and sphingolipidoses.

Sphingolipids

Sphingolipids are major components of cell membranes and are especially abundant in myelin. They are similar to the glycerol-containing phospholipids described above, except that their hydrophilic "backbone" is **serine** (Fig. 36.2 *opposite*). They are derived from **sphingosine**, which is formed when palmitoyl CoA loses a carbon atom as CO_2 in a reaction with serine. Sphingosine is *N*-acylated to form **ceramide**, which is the group common to the sphingolipids, e.g. **sphingomyelin** and the carbohydrate-containing **cerebrosides** and **gangliosides**. The **sphingolipidoses** are a group of lysosomal disorders characterised by impaired breakdown of the sphingolipids (Fig. 36.3). The lipid products that accumulate cause the disease.

Sphingomyelin

The addition of phosphorylcholine to ceramide produces **sphingomyelin** (Fig. 36.2). Sphingomyelin (also known as ceramide phosphorylcholine) is analogous to phosphatidylcholine.

Cerebrosides

When ceramide combines with a monosaccharide such as **galactose** (**Gal**) or **glucose** (**Glc**), the product is a **cerebroside**, e.g. **galactocerebroside** (or galactosylceramide) (Fig. 36.2) or **glucocerebroside** (or glucosylceramide). Cerebrosides are also known as "**mono**glycosylceramides". **Globosides** are cerebrosides containing two or more sugars.

Gaucher's disease

Gaucher's disease, the most prevalent lysosomal storage disease, is an autosomal recessive disorder caused by lysosomal deficiency of **β-glucocerebrosidase** (**GBA**) (Fig. 36.3). This results in excessive accumulation of glucocerebroside in the brain, liver, bone marrow and spleen. Type 1 Gaucher's disease (non-neuronopathic form) can be treated by **enzyme replacement therapy** (**ERT**) with recombinant β-glucocerebrosidase. In the future, Gaucher's disease is a potential candidate for gene therapy by inserting the GBA gene into haemopoietic stem cells.

Gangliosides and globosides

When ceramide combines with **oligosaccharides** and ***N*-acetylneuraminic** acid (**NANA**, also known as **sialic acid**), the **gangliosides** are formed. Gangliosides comprise approximately 5% of brain lipids.

Fabry's disease

Fabry's disease is a rare X-linked lysosomal disorder caused by deficiency of α-**galactocerebrosidase A** (Fig. 36.3). This results in the accumulation of globoside **ceramide trihexoside** (**CTH**, also known as **globotriaosylceramide**) throughout the body causing progressive renal, cardiovascular and cerebrovascular disease. Since 2002 enzyme replacement therapy using recombinant α-galactocerebrosidase has been available.

Phospholipids II: micelles, liposomes, lipoproteins and membranes

37

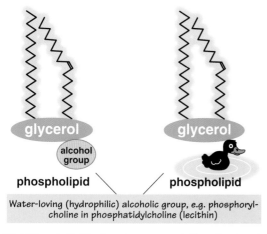

Figure 37.1 **Phospholipids**. A cartoon representation of a phospholipid is shown in which the **hydrophilic** (**water-loving**) part of the molecule (e.g. phosphorylserine or phosphorylcholine) is represented by a water-loving duck.

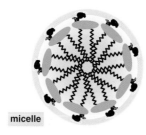

Figure 37.2 **Micelles**. When phospholipids are mixed with water they associate to form a micelle. This is a spherical structure where the **hydrophobic** parts of the molecule associate in an inner core, while the **hydrophilic** parts of the molecule associate with the surrounding water.

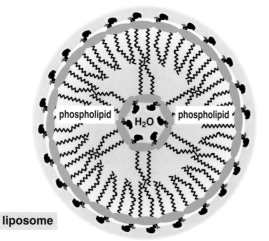

Figure 37.3 **Liposomes**. Liposomes are small artificial vesicles that are formed when phospholipids and water are subjected to high-shear mixing or to vigorous agitation by an ultrasonic probe. Liposomes can be used to encapsulate hydrophilic drugs and are used for the delivery of some anticancer drugs. They are also used to deliver cosmetics.

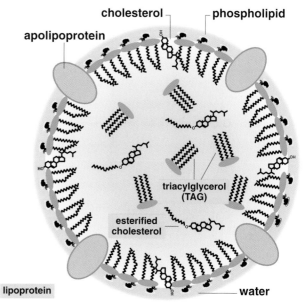

Figure 37.4 **Lipoproteins**. Lipoproteins are macromolecular complexes used by the body to transport lipids in the blood. They are characterised by an outer coat of phospholipids and proteins, which encloses an inner core of hydrophobic TAG and cholesteryl ester. Lipoproteins are classified according to the way they behave on centrifugation. This in turn corresponds to their relative densities, which depends on the proportion of (high density) protein to (low density) lipid in their structure. For example, **high density lipoproteins** (**HDLs**) consist of **50% protein** and have the highest density, while **chylomicrons** (**1% protein**) and **very low density lipoproteins** (**VLDLs**) have the lowest density.

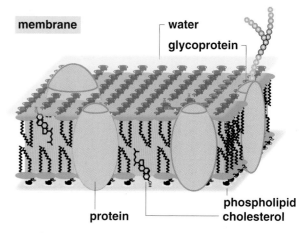

Figure 37.5 **Membranes**. The membranes in mammalian cells are composed of a mixture of phospholipids, proteins and cholesterol, which organises to form a bimolecular sheet.

Table 37.1 Apolipoproteins and their properties. The apolipoproteins are located in the outer protein-containing layer of lipoproteins. They confer on the lipoproteins their identifying characteristics.

A1	ApoA1	**In HDLs** (90% total protein) **and chylomicrons** (3% total protein) High affinity for cholesterol, removes cholesterol from cells Activates lecithin–cholesterol acyltransferase (LCAT)
B 48	ApoB48	**In chylomicrons** Made in intestine when triacylglycerol (TAG) biosynthesis is active during fat absorption
B 100	ApoB100	**In VLDLs (and in intermediate density lipoproteins (IDLs) and low density lipoproteins (LDLs), which are derived from VLDLs)** Made in hepatocytes when TAG and cholesterol biosynthesis is active Binds to receptor
C2	ApoC2	**In chylomicrons and VLDLs** Activates lipoprotein lipase when the chylomicrons and VLDLs arrive at their target tissue
E	ApoE	**In chylomicrons, VLDLs and HDLs** Binds to receptor

Table 37.2 Plasma lipoproteins. As shown in Fig. 37.4, lipoproteins are spherical structures with a **hydrophilic exterior** and a **hydrophobic** (lipid-containing) **core**. Their function is to transport lipids in the hydrophilic environment of the blood. The outer surface of lipoproteins is rich in phospholipids and apolipoproteins (Table 37.1) which confer upon the lipoproteins many of their specific properties.

Plasma lipoproteins					
	Chylomicron	Very low density lipoprotein (VLDL)	Intermediate density lipoprotein (IDL)	Low density lipoprotein (LDL)	High density lipoprotein (HDL)
Origin	Intestine	Liver	Derived from VLDLs	Derived from VLDLs and IDLs	Intestine and liver
Function	Transport dietary TAG and cholesterol from the intestines to the periphery	Forward transport of endogenous TAG and cholesterol from liver to periphery	Precursor of LDLs	Cholesterol transport	1 Reverse transport of cholesterol from periphery to the liver 2 Stores apoprotein C2 and apoprotein E which it supplies to chylomicrons and VLDLs 3 Scavenges and recycles apolipoproteins released from chylomicrons and VLDL following lipoprotein lipase activity in the capillaries
Components of lipoproteins (%)					
TAG	90	65	30	10	2
Cholesterol/ester	5	13	40	45	18
Phospholipids	4	12	20	25	30
Proteins	1	10	10	20	50
Laboratory results					
Fasting TAG (triglycerides)	Desirable: <1.5 mmol/l (<133 mg/dl)				
Total cholesterol	Target: <4.0 mmol/l (<155 mg/dl) Desirable: <5.2 mmol/l (<200 mg/dl)				
LDL cholesterol			Optimal: 2.6 mmol/l (100 mg/dl)		
HDL cholesterol					Average risk (male): 1.0–1.3 mmol/l (40–50 mg/dl) Average risk (female): 1.3–1.5 mmol/l (50–59 mg/dl)

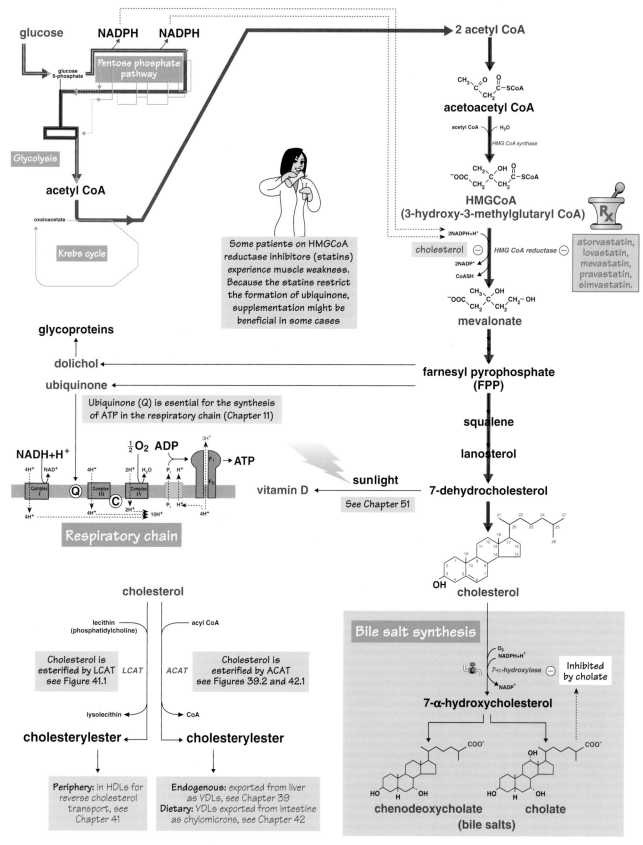

Figure 38.1 Metabolism of carbohydrate to cholesterol.

Cholesterol: friend or foe?

Cholesterol is a lipid named from the Greek roots *chole* (bile), *ster* (solid) and **ol** (because it has an alcohol group). It is normally found in bile, but if present at supersaturated concentrations it crystallises out to form "solid bile", i.e. gall stones. Cholesterol has many important functions, for example it is a **component of cell membranes**, and is a precursor of the **bile salts** (Fig. 38.1) and the steroid hormones (**aldosterone, cortisol, testosterone, progesterone** and **oestrogens** (Chapter 43)). However, if present in excessive amounts in the blood, cholesterol is deposited in arterial walls causing atherosclerosis. Cholesterol can also be deposited as yellow deposits in soft tissues causing tendon xanthomata (Greek *xantho-*, yellow), palmar xanthomata, xanthelasmata and corneal arcus.

Biosynthesis of cholesterol

Cholesterol can be made *de novo* from dietary carbohydrate

Cholesterol is made in the liver from glucose via the pentose phosphate pathway (which generates NADPH) and glycolysis, which produces acetyl CoA (Fig. 38.1). Acetyl CoA is then metabolised to **3-hydroxy-3-methylglutaryl CoA** (**HMGCoA**) which is reduced by NADPH in the presence of **HMGCoA reductase** (the regulatory enzyme for cholesterol synthesis) to form **mevalonate**. Mevalonate is then metabolised via more than two dozen intermediates (not shown) to form cholesterol.

HMGCoA reductase regulates cholesterol biosynthesis

Clearly, cholesterol biosynthesis must be regulated to prevent the diseases associated with **hypercholesterolaemia** and the regulation of HMGCoA reductase has been the subject of much research. Three mechanisms are used: (i) HMGCoA reductase is down-regulated by cholesterol (**feed-back inhibition**), (ii) insulin stimulates **HMGCoA reductase** while glucagon inhibits it (both hormonal effects are mediated by **protein phosphorylation cascades** similar to those used to regulate glycogen metabolism (Chapters 27, 31)), and (iii) cholesterol **restricts transcription** thereby decreasing the formation of mRNA needed for synthesis of HMGCoA reductase (Chapter 31).

Pharmacological treatment of hypercholesterolaemia using statins

The **statins** are reversible inhibitors of HMGCoA reductase and inhibit cholesterol biosynthesis. The resulting fall in cellular cholesterol concentration increases expression of low density lipoprotein (LDL) receptors, therefore more LDL cholesterol is removed from the blood. By lowering blood concentrations of LDL cholesterol, statins have made a dramatic impact on the prevention of cardiovascular disease. NB The statins restrict the formation of **mevalonate** and, consequently, the formation of all other downstream intermediates involved in cholesterol biosynthesis might also be restricted. In particular, the production of **farnesyl pyrophosphate** and its product **ubiquinone** will be decreased. Since ubiquinone is an essential component of the respiratory chain (Chapters 11–13), which is needed for ATP biosynthesis, it is possible that the statins could compromise the ATP production needed for energy metabolism in exercising muscle. This could be responsible for the muscle cramps or weakness experienced by some patients treated with statins and it has been suggested these patients might benefit from supplementation with ubiquinone (also known as coenzyme Q_{10}).

Ubiquinone, dolichol and vitamin D are important by-products of the cholesterol biosynthetic pathway

It has been mentioned above that **ubiquinone** is an important by-product of cholesterol biosynthesis. However, note that other by-products are **dolichol** (needed for glycoprotein biosynthesis) and **vitamin D** (Chapter 51).

Forward transport of cholesterol from the liver to peripheral tissues

Once cholesterol has been made in the liver, it must be transported to the periphery where it is needed. However, since it is not soluble in the aqueous environment of the blood it must be packaged in **v**ery **l**ow **d**ensity lipoproteins (**VLDL**s) for transport to the tissues (Chapter 39). *NB Dietary cholesterol is similarly transported from the gut in **chylomicrons** (Chapter 37 and Fig. 42.1).*

Reverse transport of cholesterol from peripheral tissues to the liver

Cholesterol is removed from peripheral tissues by high density lipoproteins (HDLs) (Chapter 41) which are frequently praised as being "good lipoproteins".

Biosynthesis of bile salts

The bile salts (**chenodeoxycholate** and **cholate**) are needed to emulsify lipids prior to intestinal absorption. Their biosynthesis from cholesterol is regulated by **7α-hydroxylase**.

39

VLDL and LDL metabolism I: "forward" cholesterol transport

Transport to and from the liver

The liver is organised into collections of cells known as lobules (Fig. 39.1). Each lobule receives blood from two sources. Like other organs, it receives oxygenated blood (via the hepatic artery). However, it also receives the venous blood that drains from the gut. The liver is unique in having an afferent venous supply, namely via the hepatic portal vein. This vein transports many products of digestion such as glucose from the gut to the liver. (**NB Chylomicrons are not transported via the portal vein**. They proceed via the **lymphatic system** before entering the thoracic duct and joining the blood stream.) The products of liver metabolism leave by two routes. Most products leave by the **hepatic vein**, which is in the centre of a liver lobule. However, certain products such as the bile salts are excreted via the **bile ducts**.

Cholesterol synthesis and transport

Cholesterol is synthesised from glucose by the liver (Chapter 38). Some of the cholesterol is esterified with fatty acids in a reaction catalysed by **a**cyl CoA–cholesterol–**a**cyl **t**ransferase (**ACAT**) to form **cholesteryl ester** (Fig. 39.2). This is hydrophobic and with its hydrophobic associate, the triacylglycerols, is stored in the core of the **nascent VLDL** particles. The nascent VLDLs leave the liver via the hepatic vein and progress to the periphery. In the peripheral capillaries, lipoprotein lipase removes much of the triacylglycerol content by

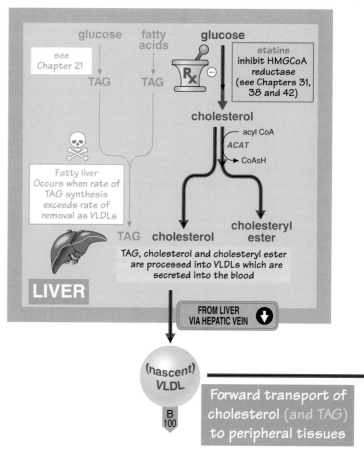

Figure 39.2 "Forward transport" of cholesterol to the peripheral tissues and its excretion as bile salts.

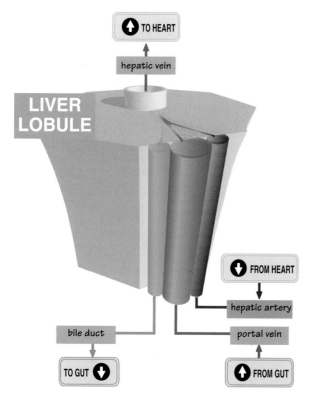

Figure 39.1 Blood enters the liver lobules via the hepatic artery and the portal vein. It leaves via the hepatic vein.

hydrolysing them to fatty acids and glycerol, leaving the remnant of the VLDL known as an **intermediate density lipoprotein** (**IDL**), which is relatively rich in cholesterol. Removal of apoE produces LDL particles which are cleared by binding to the LDL receptor. Here they are degraded to their constituent components. The cholesterol produced can be cleared from the body by conversion to bile salts (Chapter 38) which are excreted from the liver via the bile duct into the intestine. A substantial proportion of the bile salts is reabsorbed and recirculated via the liver in the "**enterohepatic circulation**".

Disorder of LDL metabolism

Type 2 hyperlipidaemia

Patients with **familial hypercholesterolaemia** have very high serum cholesterol concentrations. They die at a young age from ischaemic heart disease if they are not treated. The disorder is due to failure to produce functional **LDL receptors**. The deficit of LDL receptors results in a failure to clear LDL from the blood. The LDLs accumulate and cause atherosclerosis.

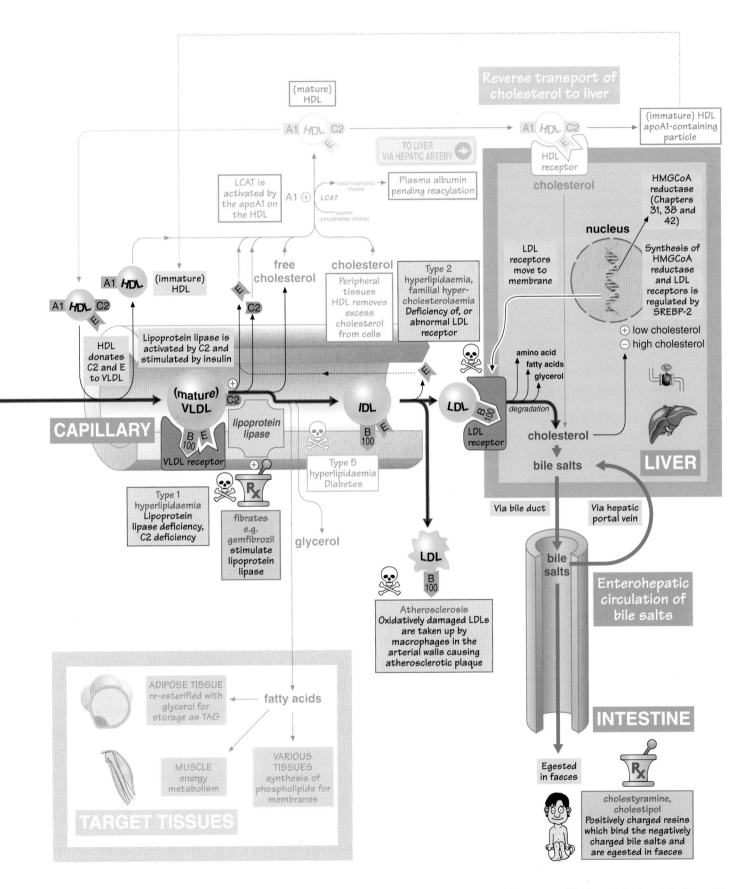

40

VLDL and LDL metabolism II: endogenous triacylglycerol transport

Biosynthesis of triacylglycerols (TAGs) in liver

We have seen in Chapter 21 how glucose can be metabolised to fatty acids. In addition to this *de novo* lipogenesis, fatty acids are also supplied from adipose tissue or as dietary fatty acids in chylomicron remnants (Fig. 40.1). The fatty acids are then esterified to form TAGs. The newly formed TAGs must not be allowed to accumulate in the liver (otherwise a fatty liver results as when geese are force-fed to make *pâté de foie gras*). The hydrophobic globules of fat must be transported in the aqueous environment of the blood. This is done by enveloping them with a hydrophilic coat of phospholipids and protein to form nascent **v**ery **l**ow **d**ensity **l**ipoproteins (**VLDLs**). The VLDLs leave the liver via the hepatic vein and are transported to the periphery.

Disposal of TAGs in target tissues

The **nascent VLDLs** while *en route* to the target tissues become **mature VLDLs** after receiving from **h**igh **d**ensity **l**ipoproteins (**HDLs**) the apolipoproteins **apoC2** and **apoE**. In the capillaries of the target tissues, the apolipoproteins apoB100 and apoE bind to the VLDL receptor and C2 activates **lipo**protein **lipase** (**LPL**), which is further stimulated by insulin. LPL hydrolyses the TAG contained in the VLDLs, producing fatty acids and glycerol. Their fate depends on the target tissue: (i) **in adipose tissue** the fatty acids are re-esterified with glycerol reforming TAG for storage; (ii) **in muscle** the fatty acids could be used for energy metabolism; or alternatively (iii) **in various tissues** the fatty acids and glycerol are synthesised to phospholipids for incorporation into cell membranes.

Disposal of IDLs and LDLs

Lipoprotein lipase in the capillaries of peripheral tissues acts on VLDLs to form intermediate density lipoproteins (**IDLs**), which are metabolised to low density lipoproteins (**LDLs**). In the liver, apoB100 of LDL binds to the LDL receptors. These are internalised, and the LDLs are degraded to fatty acids, glycerol, amino acids and cholesterol within the cell.

Disorders of VLDL metabolism

Type 3 hyperlipidaemia (remnant removal disease)

Patients have yellow streaks in the palmar creases of their hand, which is pathognomic of type 3 hyperlipidaemia. This is a rare, autosomal recessive condition caused by the production of **abnormal apoE molecules**. Since functional apoE is needed to bind the remnants of VLDL and chylomicrons to the receptor for catabolism, the remnant particles of IDLs accumulate. Laboratory tests reveal a "**broad β-band**" on electrophoresis.

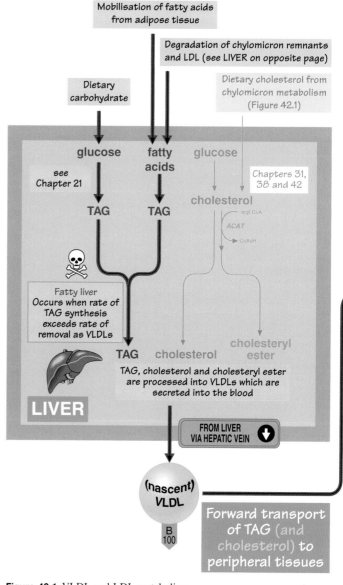

Figure 40.1 VLDL and LDL metabolism.

Type 4 hyperlipidaemia

This is an autosomal dominant dyslipidaemia characterised by overproduction of TAGs and consequently VLDLs. Serum cholesterol concentrations are normal or slightly raised.

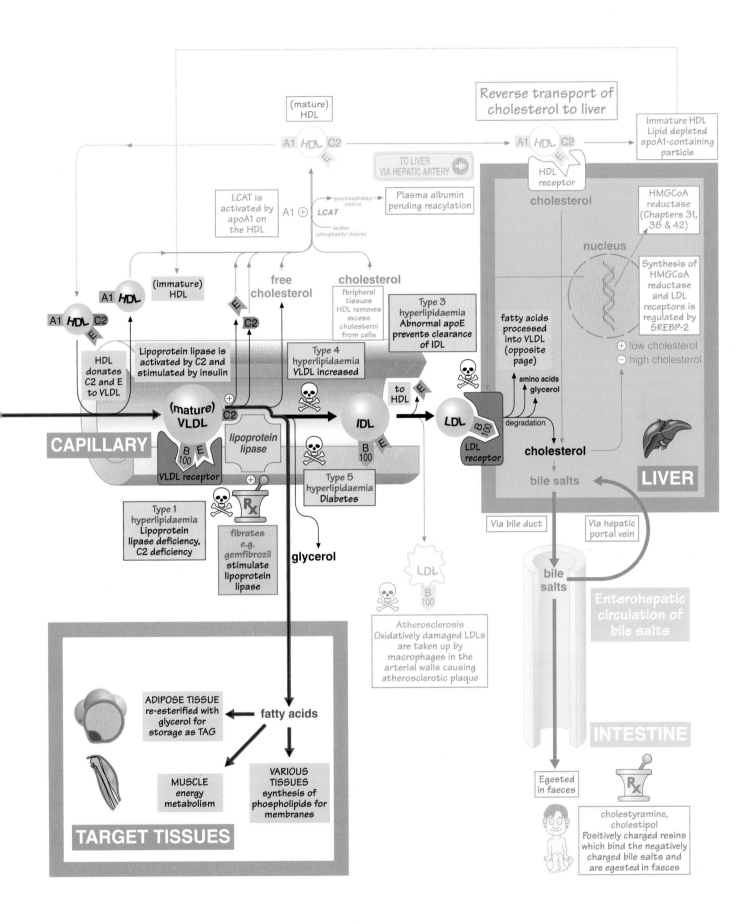

HDL are the "good" lipoproteins that dispose of excess cholesterol

The cholesterol-rich LDL particles are notorious as the "bad guys" of lipoprotein metabolism. On the other hand, HDL particles enjoy the reputation as the "good guys". This is because the function of HDL is to remove surplus cholesterol and transport it to the liver for disposal as bile salts.

HDL scavenges cholesterol from two sources:

1 Lipoprotein lipase activity primarily hydrolyses the triacylglycerol content of lipoproteins to form fatty acids and glycerol. However, in the process it liberates some cholesterol which is incorporated into HDL particles and is transported to the liver for disposal.

2 ABC transporter proteins are a ubiquitous family of proteins characterised by an **A**TP-**b**inding **c**assette (**ABC**) motif (Chapter 42). These ATP-binding proteins belong to one of the largest families known to medical science. The bound ATP is hydrolysed in a process coupled to transport of their substrate. One such protein is the cholesterol transporter known as **ABC-A1** (not shown in Fig. 41.1). It is found in many tissues where its function is to transfer excess cholesterol to HDL particles. The HDL particles proceed to the liver for disposal.

Disposal of cholesterol as bile salts

Cholesterol is metabolised to form **bile salts** (Chapter 38) which are excreted in the bile duct. The bile salts emulsify fats in the intestine, which renders them available for hydrolysis by pancreatic lipase, which is secreted into the gut. About 95% of the bile salts are absorbed into the hepatic portal vein and are recycled to the liver by the "**enterohepatic circulation**". About 5% of the bile salts are lost in the faeces.

The enterohepatic circulation can be interrupted by anticholesterol agents. These are positively charged resins that bind to the negatively charged bile salts. The resin/bile salt complex is egested in the faeces.

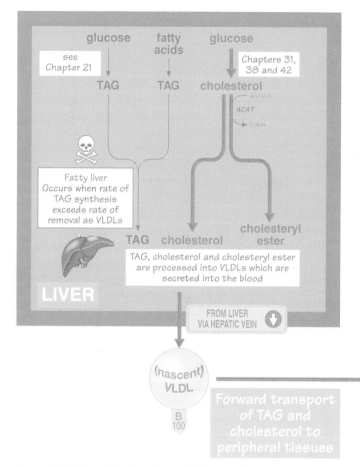

Figure 41.1 HDL metabolism: "reverse" cholesterol transport.

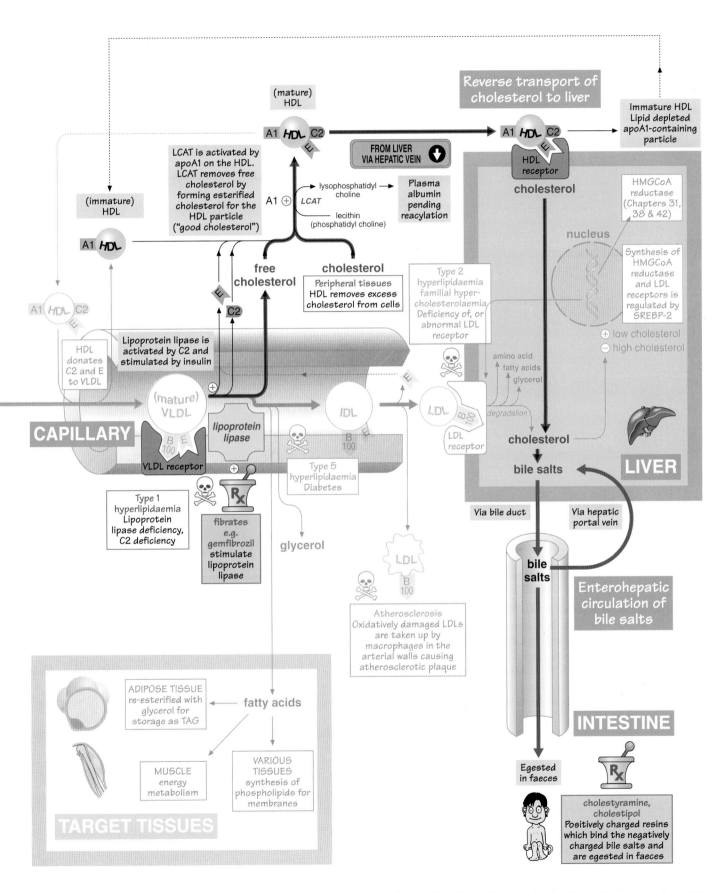

(mature)
HDL

A1 **HDL** C2
E

Reverse transport of cholesterol to liver

Immature HDL Lipid depleted apoA1-containing particle

A1 **HDL** C2
E

HDL receptor

LCAT is activated by apoA1 on the HDL. LCAT removes free cholesterol by forming esterified cholesterol for the HDL particle ("good cholesterol")

FROM LIVER VIA HEPATIC VEIN

cholesterol

A1 ⊕ *LCAT*

lysophosphatidyl choline

Plasma albumin pending reacylation

lecithin (phosphatidyl choline)

HMGCoA reductase (Chapters 31, 38 & 42)

nucleus

Synthesis of HMGCoA reductase and LDL receptors is regulated by SREBP-2

(immature) HDL

A1 **HDL**

free cholesterol

cholesterol

Peripheral tissues HDL removes excess cholesterol from cells

Type 2 hyperlipidaemia familial hyper-cholesterolaemia Deficiency of, or abnormal LDL receptor

⊕ low cholesterol
⊖ high cholesterol

A1 **HDL** C2
E

HDL donates C2 and E to VLDL

Lipoprotein lipase is activated by C2 and stimulated by insulin

E

C2

⊕

amino acid
fatty acids
glycerol

degradation

CAPILLARY

(mature) VLDL
B E 100

lipoprotein lipase

VLDL receptor

⊕
Rx

Type 1 hyperlipidaemia Lipoprotein lipase deficiency, C2 deficiency

fibrates e.g. gemfibrozil stimulate lipoprotein lipase

IDL
B 100
E

Type 5 hyperlipidaemia Diabetes

E

LDL B 100

LDL receptor

cholesterol

bile salts

LIVER

Via bile duct

Via hepatic portal vein

bile salts

glycerol

LDL B 100

Atherosclerosis Oxidatively damaged LDLs are taken up by macrophages in the arterial walls causing atherosclerotic plaque

Enterohepatic circulation of bile salts

ADIPOSE TISSUE re-esterified with glycerol for storage as TAG

fatty acids

MUSCLE energy metabolism

VARIOUS TISSUES synthesis of phospholipids for membranes

TARGET TISSUES

INTESTINE

Egested in faeces

Rx

cholestyramine, cholestipol Positively charged resins which bind the negatively charged bile salts and are egested in faeces

42 Absorption and disposal of dietary triacylglycerols and cholesterol by chylomicrons

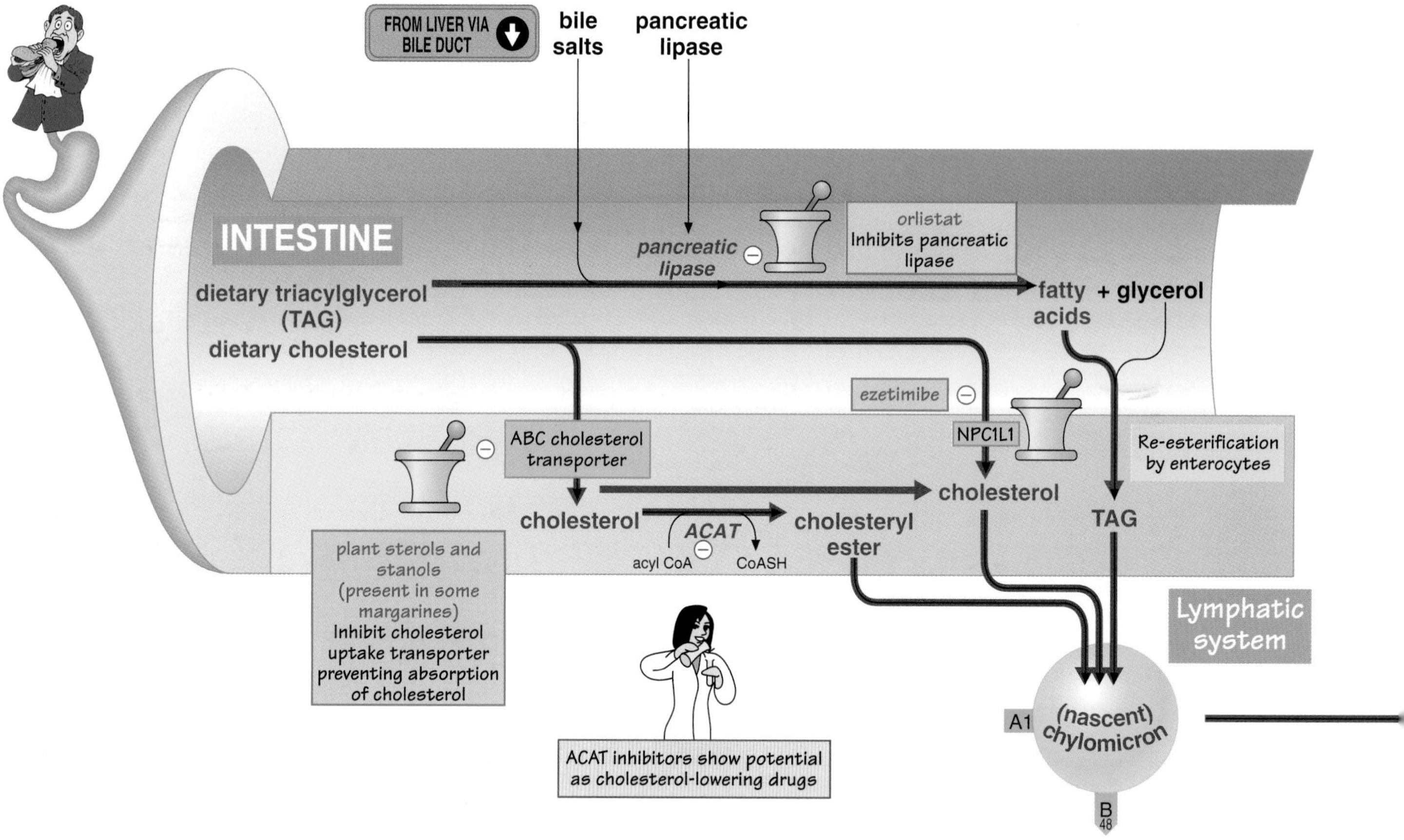

Figure 42.1 Absorption and disposal of dietary triacylglycerol and cholesterol by chylomicrons.

Absorption of dietary triacylglycerols

Dietary triacylglycerols pass through the stomach to the gut where they are emulsified in the presence of the bile salts. Pancreatic lipase is secreted into the gut where it hydrolyses triacylglycerols to fatty acids and glycerol. The fatty acids and glycerol are absorbed by the intestinal cells and re-esterified to triacylglycerols.

Intestinal absorption of cholesterol

Dietary cholesterol is absorbed by **intestinal ABC cholesterol transporter** (Chapter 41). Once inside the cell, cholesterol is esterified by **a**cyl CoA–**c**holesterol–**a**cyl **t**ransferase (**ACAT**) to form the **hydrophobic** cholesteryl ester. This reaction facilitates and maximises absorption of cholesterol, which is probably an advantage to people deprived of cholesterol-rich food such as meat. Unfortunately, efficient absorption of cholesterol is not an advantage to the affluent. However, margarines enriched with plant sterols have been used to inhibit cholesterol absorption in an attempt to lower blood cholesterol. Research is under way to develop **ACAT inhibitors** that potentially are cholesterol-lowering drugs. Ezetimibe is a new drug that inhibits cholesterol absorption by inhibition of the intestinal cholesterol-transporter protein NPC1L1 (Niemann–Pick C1-like protein 1).

For an authoritative review of lipoprotein metabolism (Chapters 35–42) see: Frayn KN (2010) *Metabolic Regulation: a human perspective*, 3rd edn. Wiley-Blackwell, Chichester, UK.

Chylomicrons

Triacylglycerols and cholesteryl ester are enveloped by a coat of phospholipids, **apoA1** and **apoB48** to form **nascent chylomicrons**. These are secreted by the enterocytes into the lymphatic system, which converge to form the thoracic duct. The thoracic duct joins the blood stream in the thorax at the left and right subclavian veins.

Disposal of triacylglycerols

Chylomicrons travel in the blood to the capillaries where they acquire **apoE** and **apoC2** from HDLs. On arrival at the target tissues, they bind to lipoprotein lipase and associated, negatively charged proteoglycans. Lipoprotein lipase is activated by apoC2 and hydrolyses the triacylglycerols to form fatty acids and glycerol. The fate of the fatty acids depends on the type of tissue. In adipose tissue, the fatty acids are re-esterified with the glycerol to reform triacylglycerols, which are stored until needed. In muscle, the fatty acids could be used as metabolic fuel.

Disposal of cholesterol

The disruption to the chylomicrons caused by lipoprotein lipase allows cholesterol to be released. This is scavenged by **HDLs** that transport the cholesterol for metabolism to bile salts in the liver.

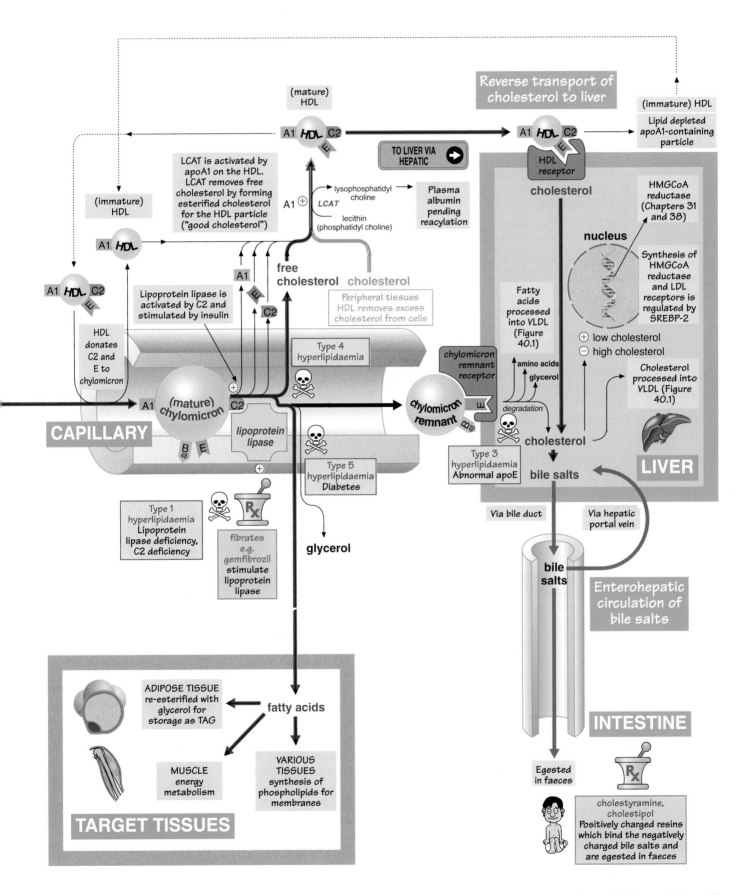

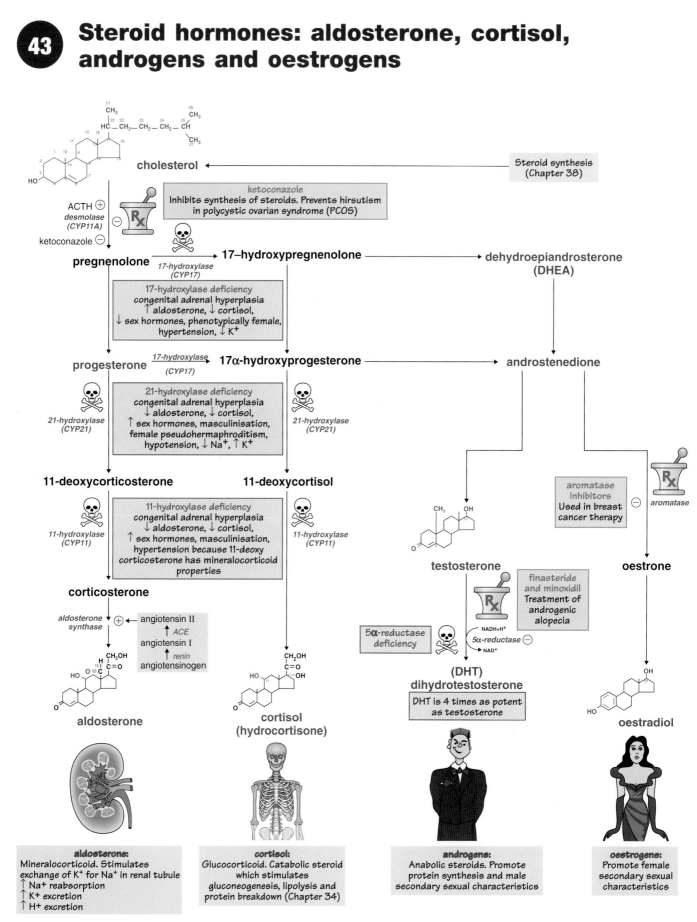

Figure 43.1 Biosynthesis of the steroid hormones.

The steroid hormones

There are four main types of steroid hormone: (i) **mineralocorticoids**, (ii) **glucocorticoids**, (iii) the male sex hormones (**androgens**), and (iv) the female sex hormones (**oestrogens**) (Fig. 43.1). NB **Androstenedione** is the precursor of **both** the androgens and oestrogens. Indeed, a wit once noted that the only difference between Romeo and Juliet was the ketone group on the 3-carbon atom and the methyl group on carbon 10 of the steroid nucleus.

Disorders of steroid hormone metabolism
Hyperaldosteronism

Conn's disease is **primary hyperaldosteronism** caused by a rare aldosterone-secreting tumour. Consequently, excessive amounts of potassium and hydrogen ions are lost in the urine resulting in hypokalaemia and metabolic alkalosis. **Secondary hyperaldosteronism** due to kidney or liver disease is more common.

Adrenocortical insufficiency (Addison's disease)

Addison's disease is a rare, potentially fatal condition due to **insufficient** production of **both aldosterone and cortisol** caused by atrophy of the adrenal glands. It is characterised by low blood pressure, loss of sodium, weight loss and pigmentation of mucosal membranes. Adrenocortical insufficiency also results from pituitary failure with loss of adrenocorticotrophic hormone (ACTH) production.

Hypercortisolism: Cushing's syndrome

Cortisol is secreted by the adrenal **cortex** in response to stress and starvation. It stimulates fat breakdown and also **glucose production** by gluconeogenesis from amino acids derived from tissue proteins. Hence cortisol is a **catabolic steroid** and is secreted during starvation. Natural steroids or synthetic analogues (e.g. dexamethasone) are known as "**glucocorticosteroids**". Secretion of cortisol is regulated by the hypothalamic/pituitary/adrenal axis that, respectively, secretes **corticotrophin-releasing hormone** (CRH) from the hypothalamus, which stimulates secretion of **ACTH** from the posterior pituitary, which stimulates secretion of **cortisol** from the adrenal cortex. Excessive amounts of cortisol cause Cushing's syndrome, which has four causes: (1) **iatrogenic**, (2) **pituitary adenoma**, (3) **adrenal adenoma/carcinoma**, and (4) **ectopic** production of **ACTH**.

1 Iatrogenic Cushing's syndrome is the most common presentation.
2 The syndrome was first described by Cushing in a patient with a rare primary pituitary adenoma that secreted ACTH. This condition is known as Cushing's disease.

3 Subsequently, patients were described with primary adrenal adenoma (benign)/carcinoma (malignant) in which blood cortisol was increased but ACTH was decreased.
4 Ectopic production of ACTH, for example by small cell lung carcinoma.

Patients with Cushing's syndrome characteristically have a moon-shaped face, thin legs and arms, and truncal obesity due to accumulation of visceral fat (like a pear on match sticks). At first, **accumulation of fat** in the presence of cortisol (a **catabolic** steroid) appears to be counterintuitive. However, hypercortisolism-driven gluconeogenesis increases the blood glucose concentration, which increases the secretion of insulin. In Cushing's syndrome, cortisol overwhelms insulin rendering it inefficient at reducing the blood glucose concentration. On the other hand, **insulin activity prevails in visceral adipose tissue** where it stimulates expression of **lipoprotein lipase**. This favours lipid accumulation in **visceral** rather than subcutaneous adipose tissue because of the higher blood flow and greater number of adipocytes in the former.

Sex hormones
Impaired androgen synthesis: 5α-reductase deficiency (5-ARD)

In this condition there is an impaired ability to produce **dihydrotestosterone** (**DHT**), causing an increased serum ratio of testosterone:DHT (Fig. 43.1). Because DHT is four times as potent as testosterone, genetic males with 5-ARD usually present as neonates with ambiguous genitalia and gender assignment is a major issue.

5α-reductase inhibitors

Finasteride and **minoxidil** are used to treat androgenic alopecia. Finasteride shrinks the prostate in benign prostatic hypertrophy (BPH). **Flutamide** is a testosterone receptor blocker used in prostate carcinoma.

Aromatase inhibitors: new drugs for breast cancer

Aromatase inhibitors, e.g. **anastrozole**, **letrozole** and **exemestane**, restrict the formation of oestrogens from androstenedione and are new drugs used to treat breast cancer (Fig. 43.1). In fact, clinical trials of letrozole were so effective that the trials were stopped as it was considered unethical to continue with volunteers on placebo.

Urea cycle and overview of amino acid catabolism

Catabolism of amino acids produces ammonium ions (NH₄⁺)

Proteins are hydrolysed in the stomach by pepsin to form amino acids. Further hydrolysis occurs in the intestine. The amino acids are absorbed. Any amino acids in excess of those needed to replace the wear and tear of tissues, and for biosynthesis to hormones, pyrimidines, purines, etc., are used for gluconeogenesis, or for energy metabolism. However, catabolism of amino acids generates **ammonium ions (NH₄⁺)**, which are very toxic. Accordingly, NH_4^+ is disposed of by conversion to **urea** which is non-toxic and is readily excreted via the kidney.

Ammonium ions are metabolised to urea in the urea cycle

Figure 44.1 shows that catabolism of amino acids generates either NH_4^+ directly or **glutamate**, which is subsequently deaminated to form NH_4^+. Ammonium ion reacts with **bicarbonate ion (HCO_3^-)** and two molecules of **ATP** in a reaction catalysed by **carbamoyl phosphate synthetase I (CPS I)** to form **carbamoyl phosphate**. This now reacts with **ornithine** to form **citrulline** in the presence of **ornithine transcarbamoylase (OTC)**. **Aspartate** (the vehicle for the second amino group) reacts with **citrulline** to form **argininosuccinate**, which is cleaved to produce fumarate and **arginine**. Finally, the arginine is hydrolysed to form **urea** and in the process generates **ornithine** which is now available to repeat the cycle.

*NB Do not confuse the **CPS I** mentioned here with **CPS II** which is involved in the synthesis of pyrimidines (Chapter 58).*

Disorders of the urea cycle: OTC deficiency

There are several rare disorders of the urea cycle. However, the most common is **OTC deficiency**, which is an X-linked disease. In severe neonatal forms of the disease, patients rapidly die from ammonium toxicity. However, the disease is variable and some boys have mild forms of the disease. In heterozygous females, the condition varies from being undetectable to a severity that matches that of the boys.

In the 1990s, there was once considerable optimism that OTC deficiency would be an ideal candidate for liver-directed **gene therapy**. Unfortunately, a study of 17 subjects with mild forms of OTC deficiency using an **adenoviral vector** demonstrated little gene transfer and when subject 18 died following complications, the trial was abandoned.

In patients with OTC deficiency, **carbamoyl phosphate** in the presence of **aspartate transcarbamoylase** is diverted to form **orotic acid** (see pyrimidine biosynthesis, Chapter 58) which can be detected in the urine and used to assist with the diagnosis.

Creatine

Arginine is the precursor of **creatine,** which combines with ATP to form **creatine phosphate** (Chapter 10). Creatine is excreted as **creatinine**.

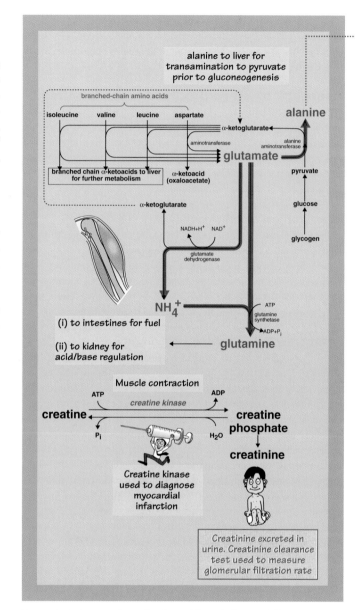

Figure 44.1 An overview of amino acid catabolism and the detoxification of NH_4^+ by forming urea.

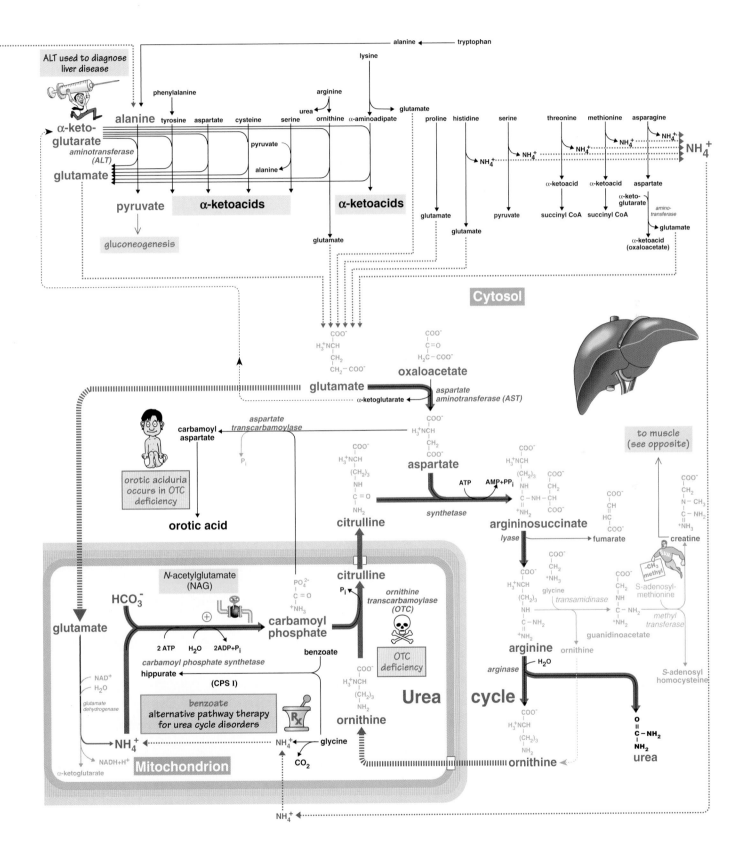

45 Non-essential and essential amino acids

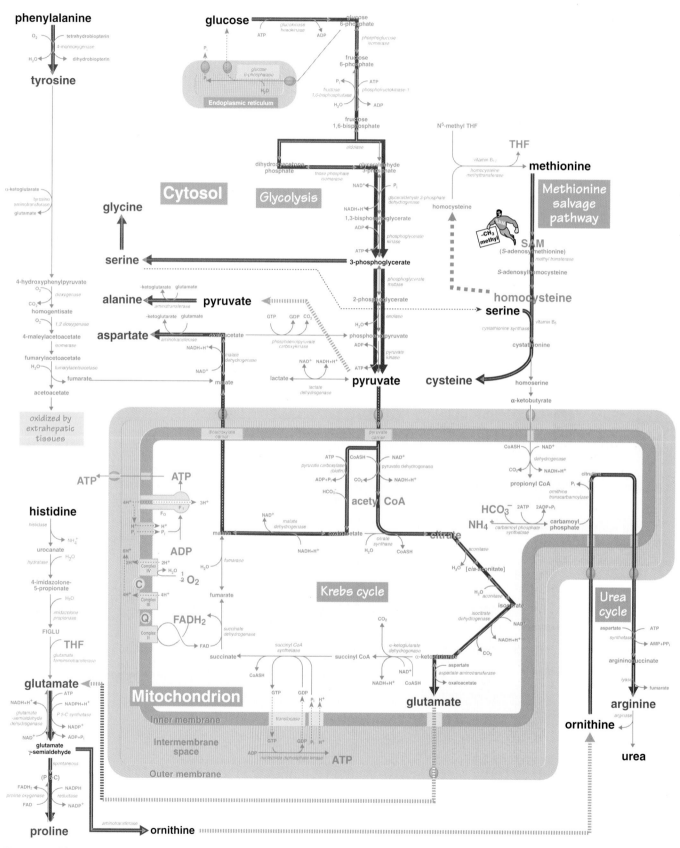

Figure 45.1 Biosynthesis of the non-essential amino acids.

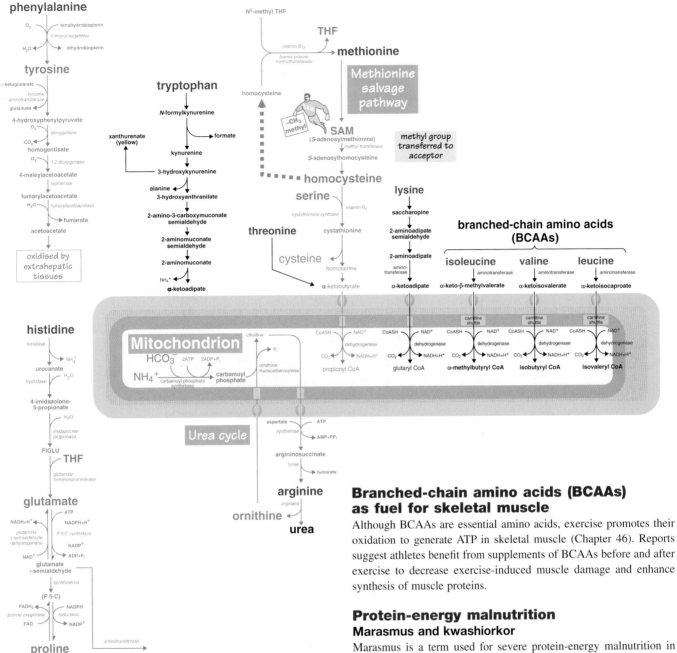

Figure 45.2 Overview of the catabolism of the essential amino acids.

Non-essential amino acids

Plants can make all the amino acids they need. However, animals (including humans) can synthesise only half the amino acids needed, namely Tyr, Gly, Ser, Ala, Asp, Cys, Glu and Pro (Fig. 45.1). These are described as **non-essential amino acids**.

Essential amino acids

Humans cannot synthesise **Phe**, **Val**, **Try**, **Thr**, **Iso**, **Met**, **His**, **Arg**, **Leu** and **Lys** (*although it is generally thought that Arg and His are only needed by children during growth periods*). Catabolism of the essential amino acids is shown in Fig. 45.2.

Branched-chain amino acids (BCAAs) as fuel for skeletal muscle

Although BCAAs are essential amino acids, exercise promotes their oxidation to generate ATP in skeletal muscle (Chapter 46). Reports suggest athletes benefit from supplements of BCAAs before and after exercise to decrease exercise-induced muscle damage and enhance synthesis of muscle proteins.

Protein-energy malnutrition
Marasmus and kwashiorkor

Marasmus is a term used for severe protein-energy malnutrition in children where the patient's weight is compared with an age-matched reference weight. Classifications vary but **normal nutrition is 90–110%** of reference weight. **Mild malnutrition is 75–90% and severe malnutrition (marasmus) is less than 60%** of reference weight matched for age.

If **oedema** is present, the malnutrition is termed **kwashiorkor** or **marasmus–kwashiorkor** if very severe.

Protein-energy malnutrition is very common in hospitalised patients, especially in the elderly, and causes difficulties with wound healing and increases pressure-sore development.

Cachexia

Cachexia is a term for extreme systemic atrophy. It generally occurs in adults where lack of nutrition causes atrophy of adipose tissue, the gut, pancreas and muscle. Cachexia is usually associated with the late stages of severe illness, especially cancer.

46 Amino acid metabolism: to energy as ATP; to glucose and ketone bodies

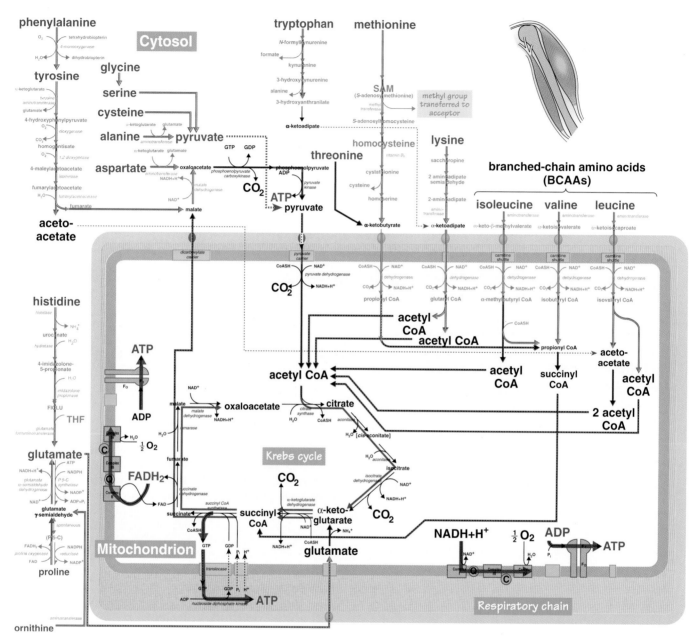

Figure 46.1 Oxidation of amino acids to provide energy as ATP in muscle.

Degradation of amino acids to provide energy as ATP

It is a common error perpetuated by most textbooks that the carbon "skeletons" derived from amino acids are oxidised when they enter Krebs cycle. **Note, that it is acetyl CoA that is oxidised to two molecules of CO₂. Therefore, before the amino acids can be fully oxidised they must be metabolised to acetyl CoA.** This is illustrated in Fig. 46.1 where the majority of amino acids enter Krebs cycle directly as acetyl CoA for oxidation to produce NADH and FADH₂, which generate ATP in the respiratory chain. *NB Certain amino acids, namely **histidine, glutamate, proline** and **ornithine**, enter Krebs cycle as α-ketoglutarate, which is **partially** oxidised to form CO₂ by α-ketoglutarate dehydrogenase. However, the remainder of the "skeleton" must leave the mitochondrion for metabolism to **acetyl CoA** prior to complete oxidation.*

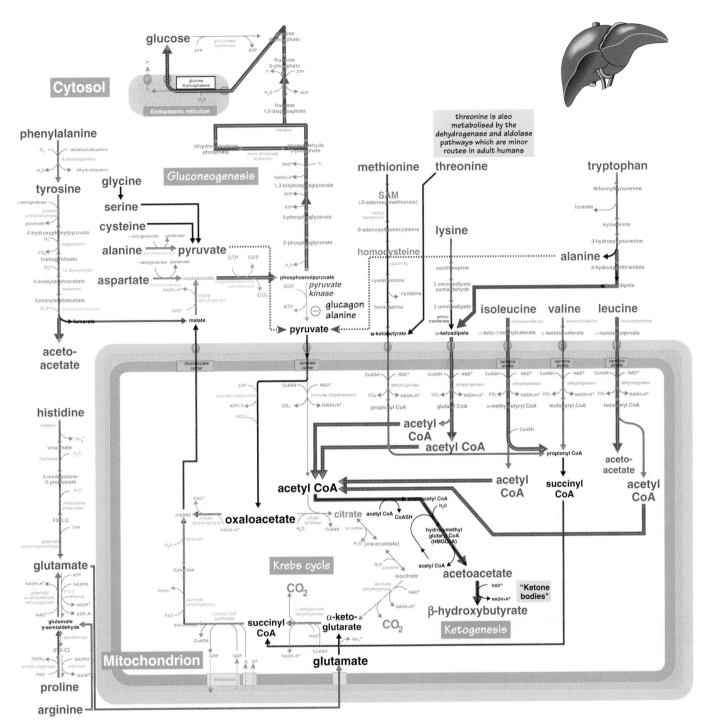

Figure 46.2 Metabolism of amino acids in fasting liver to form glucose and ketone bodies.

Metabolism of amino acids to glucose and/or ketone bodies

This is summarised in Fig. 46.2.

Glucogenic amino acids Glycine, serine, cysteine, alanine, aspartate, histidine, glutamate, proline, arginine, methionine, threonine and valine are glucogenic.

Ketogenic amino acids Lysine and leucine are ketogenic.

Amino acids that are both glucogenic and ketogenic Phenylalanine, tyrosine, isoleucine and tryptophan produce intermediates that can be metabolised to both glucose and ketone bodies.

47

Amino acid disorders: maple syrup urine disease, homocystinuria, cystinuria, alkaptonuria and albinism

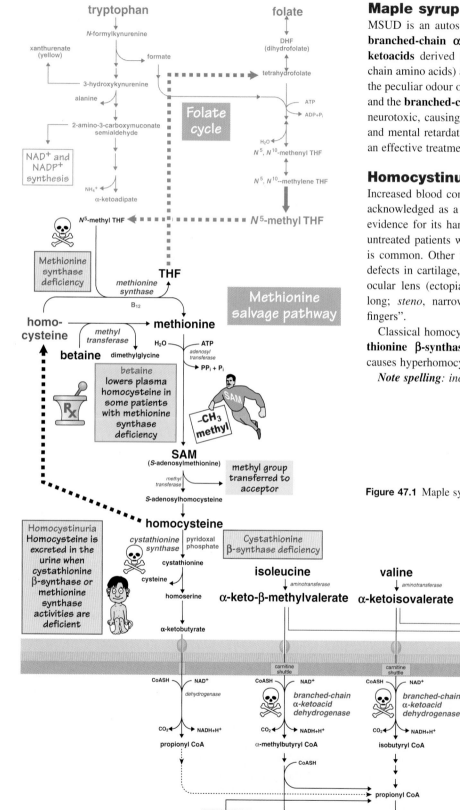

Maple syrup urine disease (MSUD)

MSUD is an autosomal recessive disorder caused by deficiency of **branched-chain α-ketoacid dehydrogenase** (Fig. 47.1). The **α-ketoacids** derived from **isoleucine**, **valine** and **leucine** (branched-chain amino acids) accumulate and are excreted in the urine, giving it the peculiar odour of maple syrup. The **branched-chain amino acids** and the **branched-chain α-ketoacids** that accumulate in the blood are neurotoxic, causing severe neurological symptoms, cerebral oedema and mental retardation. A diet low in branched-chain amino acids is an effective treatment.

Homocystinuria (HCU)

Increased blood concentrations of **homocysteine** have recently been acknowledged as a risk factor for cardiovascular disease. However, evidence for its harmful effects has been known for a long time in untreated patients with homocystinuria in whom vascular pathology is common. Other features of untreated HCU are due to structural defects in cartilage, which results in osteoporosis, dislocation of the ocular lens (ectopia lentis) and dolichostenomelia (Greek *dolicho*, long; *steno*, narrow; *melia*, limbs), otherwise known as "spider fingers".

Classical homocystinuria is caused by defective activity of **cystathionine β-synthase**. However, **methionine synthase** deficiency causes hyperhomocysteinaemia.

Note spelling: increased serum homocysteine in homocystinuria.

Figure 47.1 Maple syrup urine disease and cystinuria.

Methionine synthase deficiency

Methionine synthase is a vitamin B_{12}-dependent enzyme that needs N^5-**methyl tetrahydrofolate** (**THF**) as a coenzyme (Fig. 47.1). It catalyses the transfer of the methyl group from N^5-methyl THF to **homocysteine** to form **methionine**. When methionine synthase activity is deficient homocysteine accumulates, causing hyperhomocysti-naemia, megaloblastic anaemia and delayed development. Some patients with methionine synthase deficiency respond to supplementation with folate and vitamin B_{12}. Additional therapy using **betaine** exploits a shunt pathway that donates a methyl group to homocysteine, forming methionine.

Cystathionine β-synthase (CBS) deficiency

Cystathionine β-synthase deficiency is an autosomal recessive trait (Fig. 47.1). It is the most common cause of homocystinuria and is the second most treatable disorder of amino acid metabolism. Some patients respond to pyridoxine treatment but others are pyridoxine non-responsive. Orally administered **betaine** often lowers serum homocysteine concentrations.

Cystinuria

Cystinuria is an autosomal recessive disorder of renal tubular reabsorption of **c**ystine, **o**rnithine, **a**rginine and **l**ysine (mnemonic: **COAL**). **Cystine** (a dimer of **cysteine**; Chapter 6) is sparingly soluble and accumulates in the tubular fluid, forming bladder and kidney stones (**cystine urolithiasis**). Cystine is so-called because cystine stones were discovered in the cyst (i.e. bladder).

Alkaptonuria

Alkaptonuria is an autosomal recessive, benign disorder with a normal life expectancy. It is caused by a deficiency of **homogentisate oxidase** (Fig. 47.2). **Homogentisate** accumulates, is excreted in the urine and is gradually oxidised to a black pigment when exposed to air. It is usually detected when the nappies (or diapers) show **black staining**.

In the fourth decade signs of pigment staining appear (**onchrosis**) with slate blue or grey colouring of the ear cartilage.

Albinism (oculocutaneous albinism)

Albinism is a disorder of the synthesis or processing of the skin pigment **melanin** (Fig. 47.2). **Oculocutaneous albinism type 1** (**OCA type 1**) is an autosomal recessive disorder of **tyrosinase** resulting in the complete absence of pigment from the hair, eyes and skin. The lack of melanin in the skin makes patients with OCA type 1 vulnerable to skin cancer.

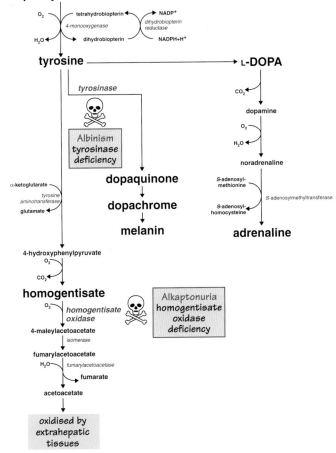

Figure 47.2 Albinism and alkaptonuria.

48

Phenylalanine and tyrosine metabolism in health and disease

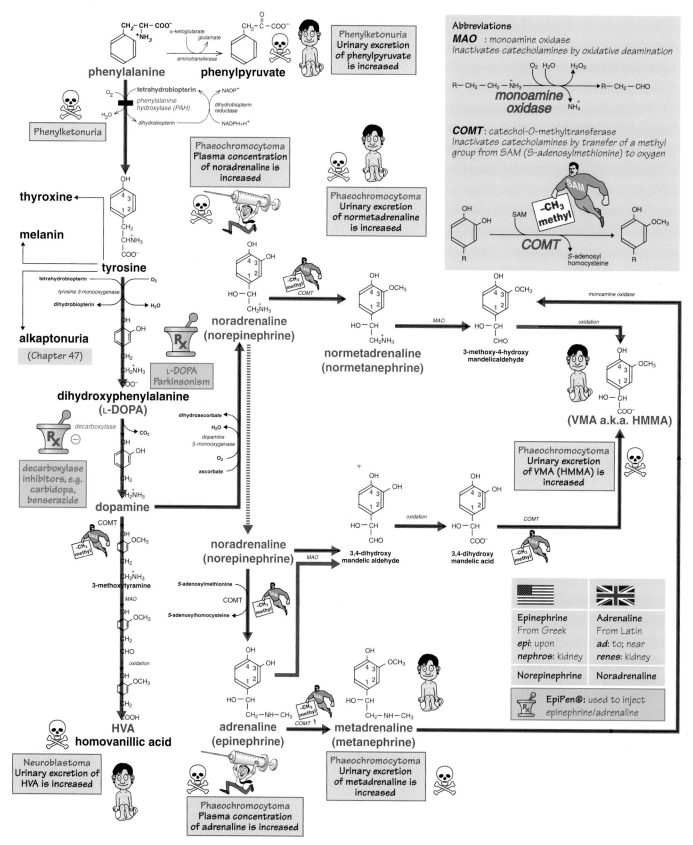

Figure 48.1 Phenylalanine and tyrosine metabolism in health and disease.

Metabolism of phenylalanine and tyrosine

Phenylalanine is an essential amino acid that can be oxidised at position 4 of the aromatic ring by **phenylalanine hydroxylase (PAH)** to form **tyrosine**. PAH (also known as phenylalanine 4-monooxygenase), needs **tetrahydrobiopterin (BH$_4$)** as a co-factor. Tyrosine is a precursor of the catecholamine hormones **dopamine**, **noradrenaline** and **adrenaline**, and also the thyroid hormone **thyroxine**. **Adrenaline** (the English name from the Latin roots that describes its anatomical relationship to the "*kidney*") has been named in their spirit of independence by our American cousins as **epinephrine** from the Greek roots meaning "*above the kidney*". The name derives from its secretion by the medulla of the adrenal gland (which is situated above the kidney) and awaits renaming by the New World as the "epinephral" gland!

Phenylketonuria (PKU)

PKU is a genetic disorder characterised by deficient metabolism of phenylalanine, resulting in the accumulation of phenylalanine and the ketone, phenylpyruvate. Neonatal screening (recently improved by the introduction of tandem mass spectrometry) for PKU assists diagnosis and treatment, which reduces the risk of mental retardation associated with this disorder.

Classic PKU Classic PKU is an autosomal recessive disease due to deficiency of **phenylalanine hydroxylase** and is treated with a low phenylalanine diet. Since phenylalanine is present in most food, dietary management is not easy, especially for a growing child. However, conscientious compliance is rewarded with a lifetime of normal achievement (Fig. 48.2).

Tetrahydrobiopterin-responsive PKU Some patients lower their blood phenylalanine in response to a **BH$_4$** loading test, particularly if the pure **6R-BH$_4$** diastereoisomer is used.

Alkaptonuria and albinism

These disorders of tyrosine metabolism are described in Chapter 47.

Metabolism of dopamine, noradrenaline and adrenaline
Biosynthesis

Tyrosine is the precursor of the **catecholamines** dopamine, noradrenaline and adrenaline. **Adrenaline** is stored in the chromaffin cells of the adrenal medulla and is secreted in the "fight or flight" response to danger. **Noradrenaline** (the "nor" prefix means it is adrenaline without the methyl group) is a neurotransmitter that is secreted into noradrenergic nerve endings. **Dopamine**, which is an intermediate in the biosynthesis of noradrenaline and adrenaline, is localised in dopaminergic neurones, notably in the substantia nigra region of the brain.

Catabolism

The major enzymes in catecholamine catabolism are **catechol-*O*-methyltransferase (COMT)** and **monoamine oxidase (MAO)**. COMT transfers a **methyl** group from *S*-**a**denosyl**m**ethionine **(SAM)** (Chapter 47) to the oxygen at position 3 of the aromatic ring (Fig. 48.1). The pathway taken is a lottery depending on whether the noradrenaline and adrenaline are first of all **methylated** (by **COMT**) or alternatively **oxidatively deaminated** (by **MAO**). If chance determines methylation has priority, then the "methylated amines" **normetadrenaline** and **metadrenaline** are formed prior to the MAO reaction and subsequent oxidation to **HMMA** (hydroxymethoxyman-

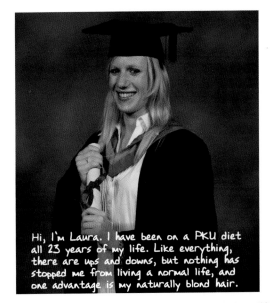

Figure 48.2 Compliance with the PKU diet is rewarded with a lifetime of normal achievement.

delic acid also known as **vanillylmandelic acid (VMA)** or **3-methoxy-4-hydroxymandelic acid (MHMA)**). On the other hand, if fate determines that the MAO reaction occurs first, then oxidation followed by methylation by COMT is the route taken to HMMA.

Catecholamine metabolism in disease
Dopamine deficiency in Parkinson's disease

In this "shaking palsy" as it was first described in 1817, the dopamine-containing neurones in the substantia nigra region of the brain degenerate. Dosing with L-**dihydroxyphenylalanine (L-DOPA)**, which crosses the **blood–brain barrier (BBB)** and is a precursor of **dopamine** (which cannot cross the BBB), provided a dramatic breakthrough in treatment. This was refined by combination with drugs such as **carbidopa** and **benserazide** (which cannot cross the BBB) as they inhibit the wasteful catabolism of L-DOPA by peripheral **decarboxylase** activity, enabling much smaller doses of L-DOPA to be used as a precursor for dopamine in the brain.

Excess adrenaline in phaeochromocytoma

A phaeochromocytoma is a rare tumour of the adrenal medulla that produces large amounts of adrenaline and/or noradrenaline. Patients suffer episodes of severe hypertension, sweating and headaches. The episodic nature of this condition means that blood and urine samples for laboratory analysis should be collected immediately after an attack as the results of tests collected between episodes are frequently normal. Laboratory investigations are urine collections for **metadrenaline**, **normetadrenaline** and **HMMA**. Sometimes, it is useful to measure blood levels of **adrenaline** and **noradrenaline**. Magnetic resonance imaging (MRI) scans locate the tumour, which can be removed by surgery.

Excessive production of dopamine

Neuroblastomas produce large amounts of dopamine anywhere in the body. They usually occur in children under 5 years old and are of neural crest cell origin. Biochemical markers are **HMMA** and the dopamine catabolic product **homovanillic acid (HVA)**.

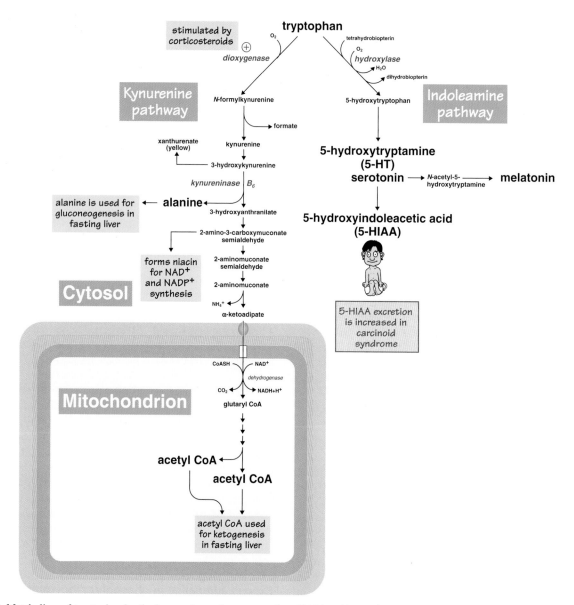

Figure 49.1 Metabolism of tryptophan by the kynurenine pathway to produce NAD⁺ and NADP⁺, or by the indoleamine pathway to produce serotonin and melatonin.

Tryptophan: the precursor of NAD⁺, NADP⁺, serotonin and melatonin

Production of NAD⁺ and NADP⁺ by the kynurenine pathway

The **kynurenine pathway** (Fig. 49.1) is the principal pathway for tryptophan metabolism and produces precursors which, together with dietary niacin, are used to synthesise **NAD⁺** and **NADP⁺** (Chapter 53). It is generally accepted that 60 mg of dietary tryptophan is equivalent to 1 mg of niacin.

Serotonin

Serotonin (5-hydroxytryptamine) is produced from tryptophan by the **indoleamine pathway**. Serotonin is important for a feeling of well-being, and a deficiency of brain serotonin is associated with depression. The **selective serotonin reuptake inhibitors** (**SSRIs**) are a successful class of antidepressive drugs that prolong the presence of serotonin in the synaptic cleft, thereby stimulating synaptic transmission in neurones that produce a sense of euphoria.

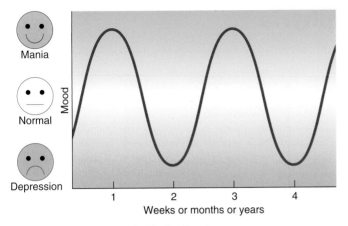

Figure 49.2 Mood changes in bipolar disorder.

Monoamine hypothesis of depression

The "monoamine hypothesis of depression" was proposed in 1965 to describe the biochemical basis of depression. Basically, it proposes that **depression** is caused by a **depletion** of monoamines (e.g. **noradrenaline** and/or **serotonin**) from the synapses. This reduces synaptic activity in the brain causing **depression**. Conversely, it suggests that **mania** is caused by an **excess** of monoamines in synapses, with excessive synaptic activity in the brain resulting in **excessive euphoria**. In **bipolar disorder**, patients have mood changes that cycle between depression and mania (Fig. 49.2).

There is evidence that systemic **corticosteroids lower serotonin** levels. This is because corticosteroids stimulate the activity of **dioxygenase**, which increases the flow of tryptophan metabolites along the **kynurenine pathway** at the expense of the **indoleamine pathway** and the production of serotonin. Lower brain concentrations of serotonin may be associated with depression. Patients with high cortisol levels (e.g. in Cushing's syndrome) are depressed, which is consistent with this hypothesis. Also, patients on a high dose regimen of steroids (e.g. prednisolone) may develop depression while on the treatment.

Carcinoid syndrome and 5-HIAA

Serotonin is metabolised to **5-hydroxyindoleacetic acid (5-HIAA)**, which is excreted in the urine. Patients with carcinoid syndrome excrete increased amounts of 5-HIAA.

Melatonin

Melatonin is made in the pineal gland and is secreted during periods of darkness. Typically, melatonin secretion begins at night-time when it aids sleeping. During daylight hours, the blood concentration of melatonin is very low.

Histamine

Histamine is involved in local immune responses and in allergenic reactions. It is also involved in controlling the amount of gastric acid produced. Histamine is produced from histidine by a decarboxylation reaction (Fig. 49.3).

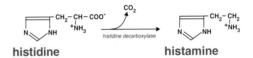

Figure 49.3 Production of histamine from histidine.

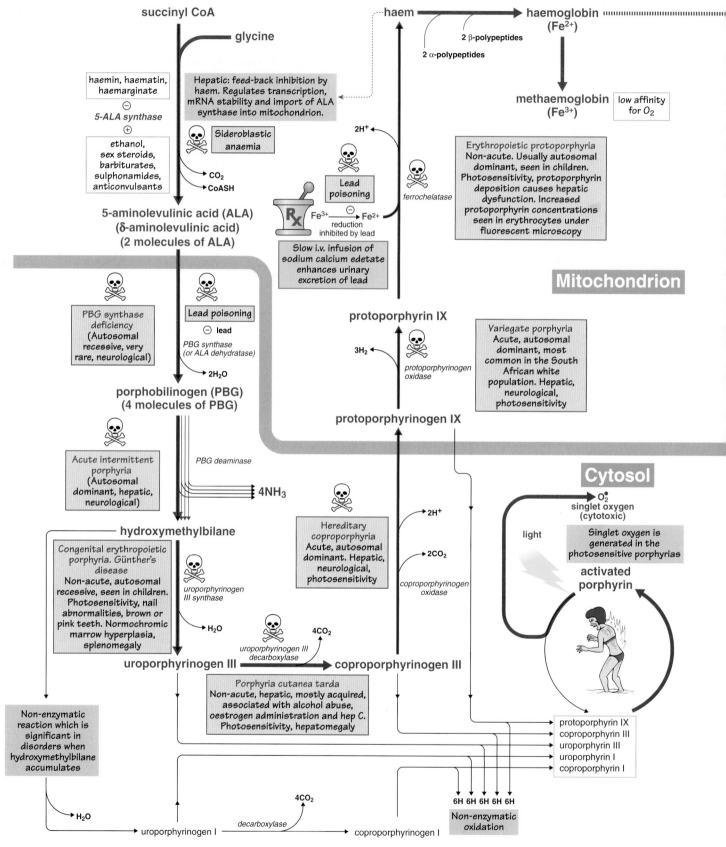

Figure 50.1 Haem, bilirubin and porphyria.

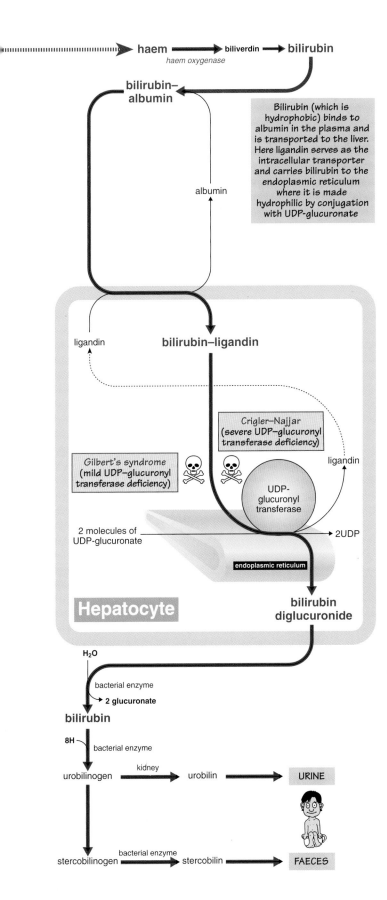

Haem biosynthesis

Haem is synthesised from **succinyl CoA** and **glycine** in most cells but particularly in liver and the haemopoietic cells of bone marrow. Hepatic haem is used to produce several haem proteins, especially the cytochrome P_{450} (CYP) family of enzymes and respiratory chain cytochromes. In erythrocytes, haem combines with globin to form haemoglobin. Haem biosynthesis is regulated by **5-aminolevulinic acid synthase** (**5-ALA synthase** also known as **δ-ALA synthase**) which, in the liver, is controlled through feed-back inhibition by haem. Hence, if the concentration of haem decreases, then 5-ALA synthase will be stimulated. The pathway also involves **porphobilinogen** (**PBG**). PBG is deaminated to form **hydroxymethylbilane**, which cyclises to **uroporphyrinogen III**, the precursor of haem (Fig. 50.1).

Acute intermittent porphyria (AIP)

This autosomal dominant condition is caused by deficiency of **PBG deaminase** and, unlike the other porphyrias, does not cause photosensitivity. The acute gastrointestinal and neuropsychiatric symptoms of AIP are caused by accumulation of 5-ALA and PBG. Episodes are triggered by ingesting alcohol and a variety of drugs, e.g. barbiturates and oral contraceptives. This is because these agents are metabolised by the cytochrome P_{450} system. Since haem is a component of cytochrome P_{450}, induction of these enzymes incorporates the available haem, consequently the haem concentration falls, the negative feedback to 5-ALA synthase is reduced and so production of PBG is enhanced. Unfortunately, because of PBG deaminase deficiency, this induced surge in **PBG accumulates** and provokes the symptoms of AIP. In AIP patients, the **urine** turns the colour of **port wine** on standing. Diagnosis is confirmed by **urine PBG excretion**. Treatment is directed at reducing 5-ALA synthase activity by intravenous infusion of haematin.

Photosensitive porphyrias

The deficiency of enzymes downstream of **hydroxymethylbilane** causes the accumulation of intermediates that are diverted by non-enzymic oxidation to form several porphyrins which, when exposed to light, form **singlet oxygen $O_2^{\cdot}$**. This is cytotoxic, causing photosensitivity on exposure to sunlight.

Lead poisoning

Lead inhibits **PBG synthase** and **ferrochelatase**, restricting haem biosynthesis and resulting in microcytic hypochromic anaemia and porphyria. Urinary excretion of 5-ALA is increased.

Haem catabolism to bilirubin

Haem is degraded by **haem oxygenase** in the reticuloendothelial system to **bilirubin**. Bilirubin is hydrophobic and is transported in the blood by albumin. In jaundice, bilirubin is produced in excess and the lipophilic bilirubin accumulates in the brain causing kernicterus. Normally, bilirubin is conjugated in the liver to **bilirubin diglucuronide**, which is water soluble and is excreted in the bile. Bilirubin diglucuronide then passes into the small intestine where bacterial enzymes produce **urobilinogen**. Urobilinogen can be absorbed and passed to the liver where it is re-excreted in the bile. A small amount, however, is excreted in urine as **urobilin**. Urobilinogen remaining in the intestine is converted to **stercobilin**, which is egested in the faeces.

Fat-soluble vitamins I: vitamins A and D

The fat-soluble vitamins A, D, E and K are absorbed by the intestines and incorporated into chylomicrons (Chapter 42). Therefore, diseases that affect fat absorption causing steatorrhoea will also affect the uptake of these vitamins. Furthermore, fat absorption relies on pancreatic lipase, which if compromised, e.g. in cystic fibrosis, can cause deficiency of one or more fat-soluble vitamins.

Vitamin A

Vitamin A is a generic term that includes "**preformed vitamin A**", namely "**retinol** (alcohol), **retinal** (aldehyde) and **retinoic acid** (carboxylic acid)", and the **provitamin A carotenoids**, which are those carotenoids capable of metabolism to retinol, e.g. β-**carotene** (Fig. 51.1).

Biochemical function

1 Vision. Retinol is metabolised to 11-*cis* retinal which binds to opsin in the rod cells forming the visual pigment "rhodopsin". A photon of light converts 11-*cis* retinal to *all-trans* retinal, initiating a series of reactions culminating in a signal to the optic nerve. This is transmitted to the brain where it is interpreted as a visual image.

2 Control of gene expression. Retinal can be oxidised to retinoic acid, which affects gene expression. Inside the nucleus, retinoic acid binds to receptors that regulate the activity of chromosomal retinoic acid response elements (RARE). By stimulating and repressing gene transcription, retinoic acid regulates the differentiation of cells and so is important for growth and development, including lymphocytes which are vital for the immune response.

Deficiency diseases

1 Vision disorders. Early vitamin A deficiency causes impaired night vision. Severe vitamin A deficiency causes xerophthalmia that progresses to corneal scarring and blindness. It occurs in over 100 million children in poor nations where rice is the staple food. Recently a form of rice rich in vitamin A ("Golden Rice") has been developed by new GM (genetic modification) technology and has the potential to prevent or reduce this tragedy.

2 Cell differentiation disorders. Vitamin A is the "anti-infection vitamin". Impaired cell differentiation caused by vitamin A deficiency impairs formation of lymphocytes and is manifest as immunodeficiency disease resulting in increased susceptibility to infectious diseases.

Dietary sources

Vitamin A is available either from: (i) **preformed retinol** (present in animal foods as retinyl esters), or (ii) metabolised from **provitamin A precursors**. The recommended dietary allowance for preformed vitamin A is 0.9 mg/day for men and 0.7 mg/day for women. Provitamin A sources are graded according to their **retinol activity equivalence** (**RAE**), e.g. since 12 mg of β-carotene in food yields 1 mg retinol, its RAE is 12.

1 Preformed vitamin A is found in liver products, fortified breakfast cereals, eggs and dairy products.

2 Provitamin A. Carotenoids are a large family of coloured compounds that are abundant in plants. About 10% of carotenoids have the β-**ionone ring**, which is needed for vitamin A activity, e.g. β-**carotene** found in carrots. Carotenoids have numerous double bonds that ensure they are efficient **free radical scavengers** and they can neutralise singlet oxygen.

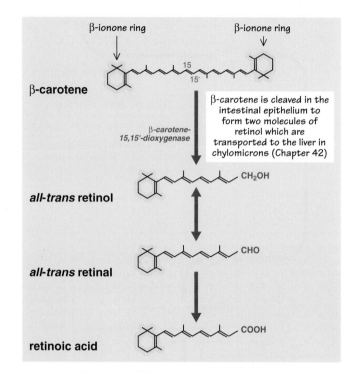

Figure 51.1 Metabolism of β-carotene to retinoic acid.

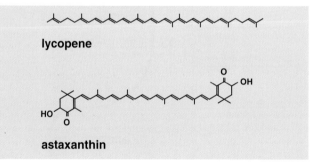

Figure 51.2 Lycopene and astaxanthin are carotenoids (but not vitamin A precursors).

Not all carotenoids are vitamin A precursors – they comprise 90% of carotenoids, nevertheless they are excellent free radical scavengers. Examples are **lycopene** (in tomatoes) and **astaxanthin** (Fig. 51.2). The latter is enjoying a reputation as a nutriceutical; it is pink and found in aquatic animals, e.g. salmon, shrimp and lobster, and in the alga, *Haematococcus pluvialis*, from which it is commercially extracted.

Toxicity

Hypervitaminosis A results from the excessive intake of preformed vitamin A. Toxicity in pregnancy is related to the role of retinoic acid in regulating differentiation, resulting in birth defects. Recent reports suggest that habitual high doses of vitamin A might be associated with osteoporosis.

Don't eat polar bear liver! 500 g of polar bear liver contains up to 10 million IU of vitamin A. Arctic explorers, their dogs and Inuit people have suffered acute vitamin A toxicity after eating it.

Vitamin A analogues

Isotretinoin and **etretinate** are analogues of vitamin A used to treat skin disorders. Isotretinoin is used to treat severe acne (but must be avoided in pregnancy, see above). Etretinate was used to treat psoriasis but it has been withdrawn in some countries.

Vitamin D

Vitamin D is the "**sunshine vitamin**". It was originally discovered as a crude mixture called **vitamin D₁** (no longer available as a supplement). **Ergosterol**, the plant equivalent of cholesterol, is converted to **vitamin D₂** by ultraviolet light. **Vitamin D₃** (**cholecalciferol**) is formed in the skin from **7-dehydrocholesterol** (an intermediate in the cholesterol biosynthesis pathway) in the presence of ultraviolet light, which opens the B-ring of the steroid nucleus (Fig. 51.3). Cholecalciferol is successively hydroxylated first in the liver forming 25-hydroxycholecalciferol (25-HCC) and then in the kidney to form the most active form: **1,25-dihydroxycholecalciferol (1,25-DHCC)**, also known as **calcitriol**.

Biochemical function

1,25-DHCC controls calcium metabolism by increasing blood calcium. It increases **intestinal** absorption of dietary calcium, in **bone** it stimulates resorption of calcium, and in the **kidney** it stimulates reabsorption of calcium into the blood.

Diagnostic tests for deficiency

Urinary calcium is low. Measure serum 25-HCC.

Dietary sources

There are few natural dietary sources, but they include fish liver oils and fatty fish (e.g. sardines, mackerel, salmon). Several foods, e.g. breakfast cereals, orange juice, margarine and milk, are fortified with vitamin D (cholecalciferol or ergocalciferol).

Deficiency diseases

Deficiency causes hypocalcaemia, resulting in rickets in children or osteomalacia in adults. Hypocalcaemic convulsions and tetany can occur.

1 Lack of sunlight. Exposure to sunlight can provide sufficient vitamin D. However, in latitudes greater than 40° north or south "vitamin D winter deficiency" can occur. People with dark skin can suffer deficiency especially if their skin is completely covered and they live in the northern or southern latitudes previously mentioned. Such people, for example Muslim women living in northern Europe, can be hypocalcaemic.

2 Malabsorption. Steatorrhoea caused by exocrine pancreatic disease or biliary obstruction can cause vitamin D deficiency.

3 Chronic renal failure. Normal kidney function is needed for the 1α-hydroxylation reaction that produces 1,25-DHCC. In chronic renal failure a cascade of events is triggered, leading to secondary hyperparathyroidism, which can progress to tertiary hyperparathyroidism and renal bone disease.

Toxicity

Hypervitaminosis D produces hypercalcaemia that can result in bone loss, organ calcification (e.g. kidneys and heart) and kidney stones.

Vitamin D hypersensitivity in sarcoidosis: extrarenal 1α-hydroxylase activity occurs in sarcoid granulomas, which converts vitamin D to inappropriately high concentrations of 1,25-DHCC, causing hypercalcaemia. Also occurs in some lymphomas and sarcomas.

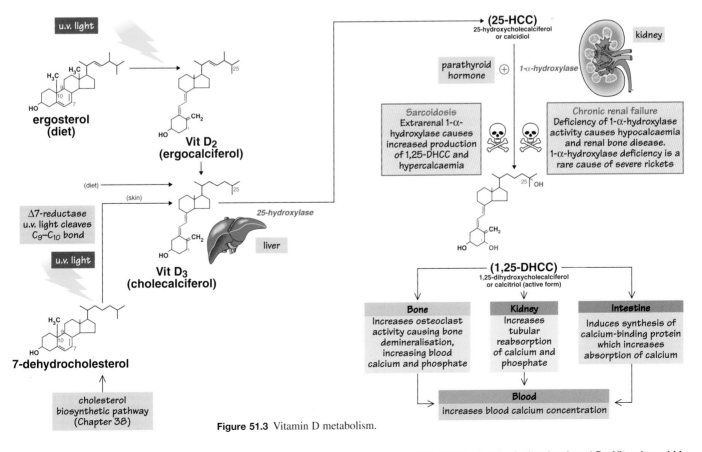

Figure 51.3 Vitamin D metabolism.

52 Fat-soluble vitamins II: vitamins E and K

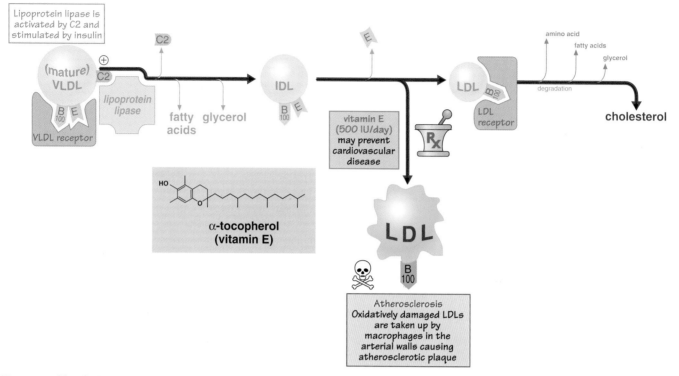

Figure 52.1 Vitamin E reduces oxidative damage to low density lipoproteins (LDLs).

Vitamin E

Vitamin E is a generic term for four tocopherols (α-, β-, γ- and δ-) and four tocotrienols (α-, β-, γ- and δ-). Of these, **α-tocopherol** is the most important.

Biochemical function

α-tocopherol is an antioxidant that prevents free radical damage to polyunsaturated fatty acids, particularly those in the cell membrane of red blood cells. Evidence suggests α-tocopherol reduces oxidative damage to low density lipoproteins (LDLs), which is associated with the development of atherosclerosis (Chapters 15, 39; Figure 52.1). Disappointingly, claims that dietary supplementation with α-tocopherol decreases cardiovascular disease are controversial. However, recent studies using 500 IU α-tocopherol/day claim inhibition of lipid oxidation in atherosclerotic lesions.

Diagnostic test for deficiency

Measure platelet vitamin E concentration.

Dietary sources

Vegetable oils, nuts and green leafy vegetables.

Deficiency diseases

Vitamin E deficiency occurs in children with cystic fibrosis and patients with steatorrhoea. Red cell membrane damage results in haemolytic anaemia. Damage to nerve cells causes peripheral neuropathy.

Toxicity

Few toxic effects have been reported, however high doses might cause increased clotting times in subjects with a low vitamin K status.

Vitamin K

Vitamin K, from the Danish *koagulation*, exists in two natural forms: **vitamin K_1 (phylloquinone)** and **vitamin K_2 (menaquinone)**. **Vitamin K_3 (menadione)** is a synthetic, water-soluble analogue.

Biochemical functions

Vitamin K is essential for activity of **vitamin K-dependent γ-glutamyl carboxylase**, which is responsible for post-translational modification of glutamyl residues (Glu) to γ-carboxylated glutamyl residues (Gla) producing a small family of **vitamin K-dependent proteins (VKD proteins)**. It is membrane bound and carboxylates the proteins as they emerge from the endoplasmic reticulum. The VKD proteins associated with blood clotting are well established but recent research has revealed VKD proteins associated with bone metabolism (bone Gla protein (BGP) and matrix Gla protein (MGP)).

1 Blood clotting. The precursors of the **anticoagulants prothrombin and factors VII, IX** and **X** are activated when **glutamate** (Glu) residues are carboxylated to γ-**carboxyglutamate** (**Gla**) by a vitamin K-dependent reaction. This process is linked to regeneration of vitamin K in the "**vitamin K epoxide cycle**" (Fig. 52.2).

2 Bone mineralisation. Recent evidence is emerging that suggests that vitamin K plays a role in bone growth and development.

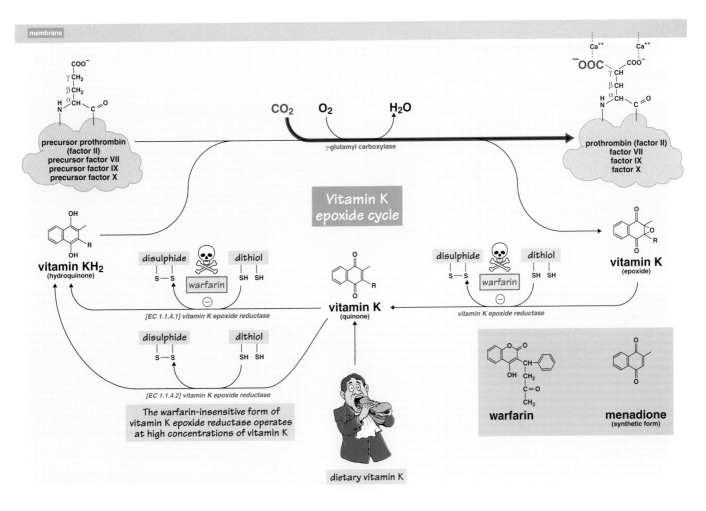

Figure 52.2 The vitamin K epoxide cycle.

Diagnostic test for deficiency

Measure undercarboxylated Gla proteins in the blood.

Dietary sources

The major source is **phylloquinone** (**vitamin K₁**) found in vegetable oils and green leafy vegetables. **Menaquinone** (**vitamin K₂**) is synthesised by the flora of the large intestine.

Deficiency diseases

1 Haemorrhagic disease of the newborn. Placental transfer of vitamin K is inefficient so deficiency can occur, resulting in neonatal haemorrhage.

2 Newborns have a sterile intestinal tract and there is therefore no bacterial source.

3 Breast milk is a poor source of vitamin K.

4 Osteoporosis. Recent research has investigated an association between osteoporotic fracture and vitamin K.

Toxicity

Toxicity with high doses of phylloquinone and menaquinone has not been reported. However, intravenous menadione causes oxidative damage to red cell membranes (haemolysis).

Water-soluble vitamins I: thiamin, riboflavin, niacin and pantothenate

53

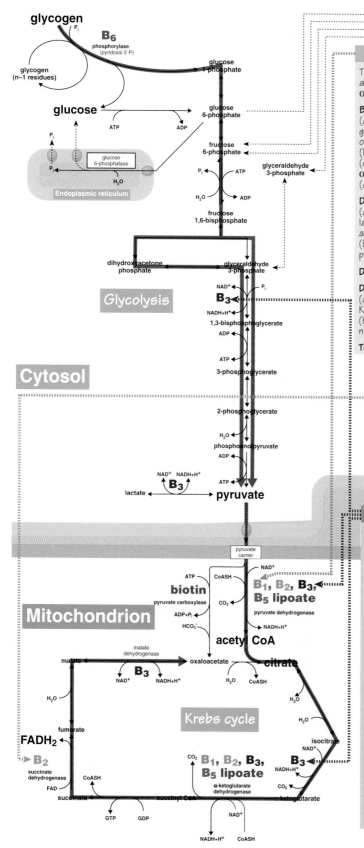

Thiamin pyrophosphate (Vitamin B₁)

Thiamin pyrophosphate (vitamin B_1) is essential for pyruvate dehydrogenase and similar large multienzyme complexes which oxidatively decarboxylate α-ketoacids. RNI 0.4 mg/1000 kcal (depends on energy intake)

Biochemical functions
(a) Cofactor for pyruvate dehydrogenase in the "link reaction" between glycolysis and Krebs cycle. Involved in energy metabolism from glucose and other carbohydrates
(b) Cofactor for α-ketoglutarate dehydrogenase
(c) Cofactor for several α-ketoacid dehydrogenases, e.g. the branched-chain α-ketoacid dehydrogenases involved in amino acid oxidation
(d) Cofactor for transketolase in the pentose phosphate pathway

Diagnostic tests
(a) Hyperlactataemia especially after a glucose load when pyruvate and lactate (which are immediately upstream of pyruvate dehydrogenase) accumulate.
(b) Measurement of red blood cell transketolase activity in the absence and presence of additional thiamin

Dietary sources: cereals, pulses, yeast, liver

Deficiency diseases
(a) Associated with alcohol abuse causing Wernicke's encephalopathy and Korsakoff's dementia
(b) Wet beriberi: oedema, cardiovascular disease; and Dry beriberi: neuropathy and muscle wasting

Toxicity: 3 g/day (variety of clinical signs)

Niacin (Vitamin B₃)

Niacin is a component of the hydrogen carriers, NAD^+ and $NADP^+$. Both have numerous roles in metabolism but NAD^+ is especially important as a "hydrogen carrier" for ATP production by the respiratory chain, whereas NADPH is very important for biosynthetic reactions. Daily requirement: 6.6 niacin equivalents/1000 kcal

Biochemical functions: niacin is a term for nicotinic acid & nicotinamide. A component of NAD^+ and $NADP^+$, and their reduced forms, NADH and NADPH which are involved in numerous metabolic reactions. NAD^+ is involved in glycolysis, the oxidation of fatty acids, amino acid oxidation and Krebs cycle. It is particularly important as a "hydrogen carrier" since oxidation of NADH by the respiratory chain generates ATP. $NADP^+$ and its reduced form $NADPH^+$ are particularly important in biosynthetic reactions, e.g. lipid synthesis.

Diagnostic test for deficiency: measure the ratio in urine of NMN/pyridone (N′-methylnicotinamide / N′-methyl-2-pyridone-5-carboximide)

Dietary sources: vitamin-enriched breakfast cereals, liver, yeast, meat, pulses. Approximately half the daily requirement can be biosynthesised from tryptophan (60 mg of tryptophan ≡ 1 mg niacin)

Deficiency diseases: pellagra (from the Italian "rough skin") occurs if diet is deficient in BOTH niacin and tryptophan such as maize-based diets (dermatitis, diarrhoea, dementia)

Pharmacology/toxicity: pharmacological doses (of 2–4 g daily) have been used in trials as a hypolipidaemic agent
Excessive nicotinic acid can cause transient vasodilation with hypotension

Figure 53.1 The role of water-soluble vitamins in metabolism.

Riboflavin (Vitamin B₂)

Riboflavin (vitamin B₂) is involved in energy metabolism from glucose and fatty acids. A component of FAD which is the prosthetic group of several enzymes used in oxidation/reduction reactions. Also a component of FMN which is in complex I of the respiratory chain

Biochemical functions: a component of FAD which is
(a) Needed for the multi-enzyme complexes involved in oxidative decarboxylation
  (i) Cofactor for pyruvate dehydrogenase in the "link reaction" between glycolysis and Krebs cycle. Cofactor for α-ketoglutarate dehydrogenase
  (ii) Cofactor for several α-ketoacid dehydrogenases, e.g. the branched-chain α-ketoacid dehydrogenases involved in amino acid oxidation
(b) Prosthetic group for succinate dehydrogenase in Krebs cycle
(c) A constituent of FMN which is a component of complex I in the respiratory chain
(d) Cofactor for acyl CoA dehydrogenase in β-oxidation

Diagnostic tests:
(a) Measure activity of red blood cell glutathione reductase which is a FAD-dependent enzyme
(b) Measure urinary secretion of riboflavin

Dietary sources: milk, liver, yeast, eggs. Present in fortified cereal products but poor in natural cereals

Deficiency diseases:
(a) Inflamed, magenta-coloured tongue.
(b) Ultraviolet light destroys riboflavin and so neonates given phototherapy for jaundice need riboflavin supplements

Toxicity: No evidence of toxicity

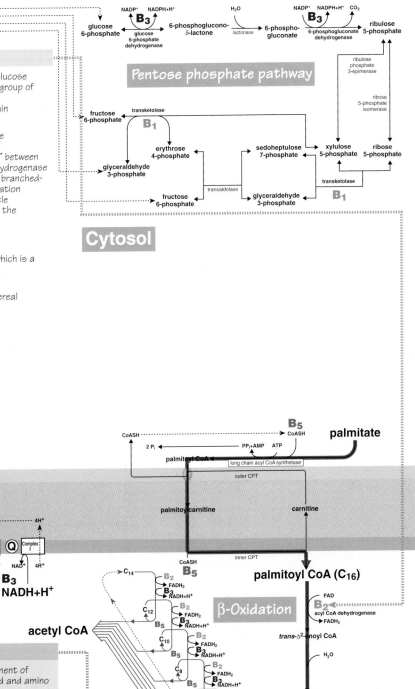

Pantothenate (Vitamin B₅)

Pantothenate (vitamin B₅) is especially important as a component of coenzyme A which has numerous functions in carbohydrate, lipid and amino acid metabolism. Daily requirement 4–7 mg

Biochemical functions: pantothenate is a component of coenzyme A (CoASH) which has numerous functions in carbohydrate, lipid and amino acid metabolism. (NB The "SH" refers to the terminal sulphydryl group in coenzyme A, Chapter 9)
Also a component of the acyl carrier protein used in fatty acid synthesis.

Diagnostic test: measure blood concentration

Dietary sources: ubiquitous, present in all foods

Deficiency diseases: apart from the infamous "burning feet syndrome" seen in prisoners of war, deficiency conditions have not been described

Toxicity: none up to 10 g/day

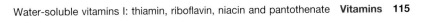

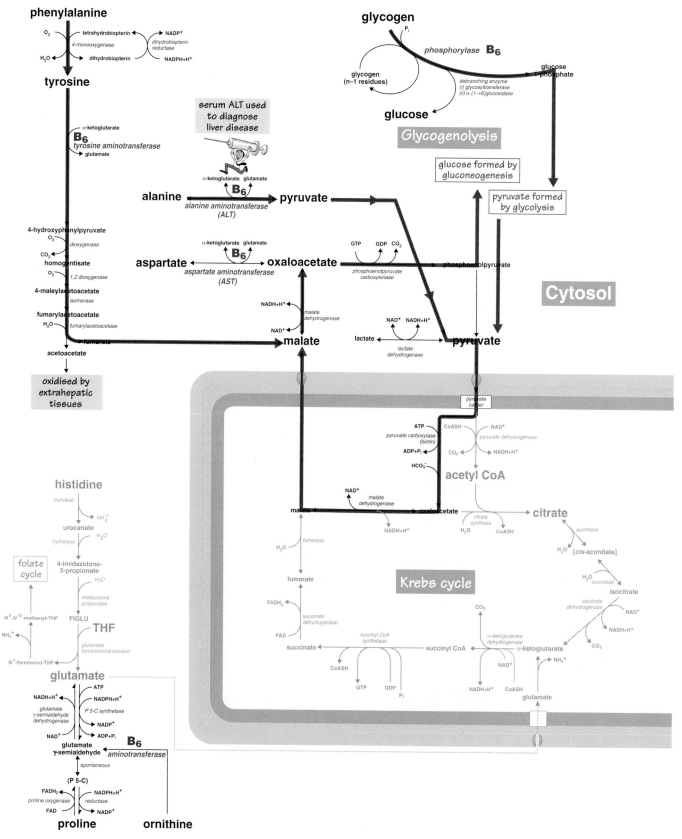

Figure 54.1 The role of vitamin B₆ in metabolism.

Transamination

Transamination is a reaction requiring vitamin B_6 (pyridoxal phosphate), which is involved in the metabolism of amino acids. Figures 54.1 and 54.2 show the transfer of amino groups from the different amino acids to α-ketoglutarate to form their respective α-ketoacids and **glutamate**. In particular, the example of **al**anine aminotransferase (**ALT**) is shown. ALT is a reversible reaction that transfers an amino group from alanine to α-ketoglutarate to form **glutamate** and **pyruvate**. ALT is used as a sensitive *"liver function test"* as it appears in the serum of patients with hepatocellular damage.

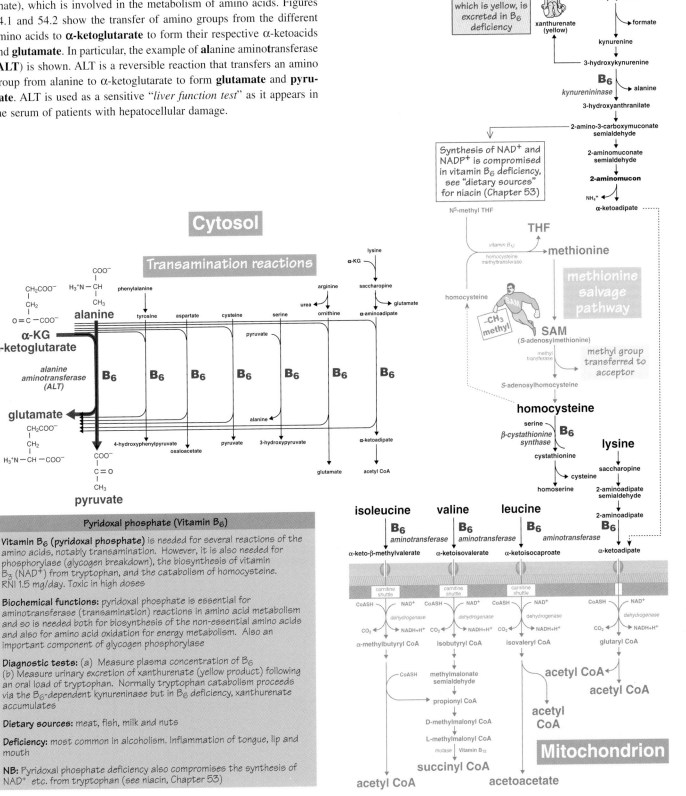

Pyridoxal phosphate (Vitamin B_6)

Vitamin B_6 (pyridoxal phosphate) is needed for several reactions of the amino acids, notably transamination. However, it is also needed for phosphorylase (glycogen breakdown), the biosynthesis of vitamin B_3 (NAD⁺) from tryptophan, and the catabolism of homocysteine. RNI 1.5 mg/day. Toxic in high doses

Biochemical functions: pyridoxal phosphate is essential for aminotransferase (transamination) reactions in amino acid metabolism and so is needed both for biosynthesis of the non-essential amino acids and also for amino acid oxidation for energy metabolism. Also an important component of glycogen phosphorylase

Diagnostic tests: (a) Measure plasma concentration of B_6
(b) Measure urinary excretion of xanthurenate (yellow product) following an oral load of tryptophan. Normally tryptophan catabolism proceeds via the B_6-dependent kynureninase but in B_6 deficiency, xanthurenate accumulates

Dietary sources: meat, fish, milk and nuts

Deficiency: most common in alcoholism. Inflammation of tongue, lip and mouth

NB: Pyridoxal phosphate deficiency also compromises the synthesis of NAD⁺ etc. from tryptophan (see niacin, Chapter 53)

Figure 54.2 The role of vitamin B_6 in metabolism (*continued*).

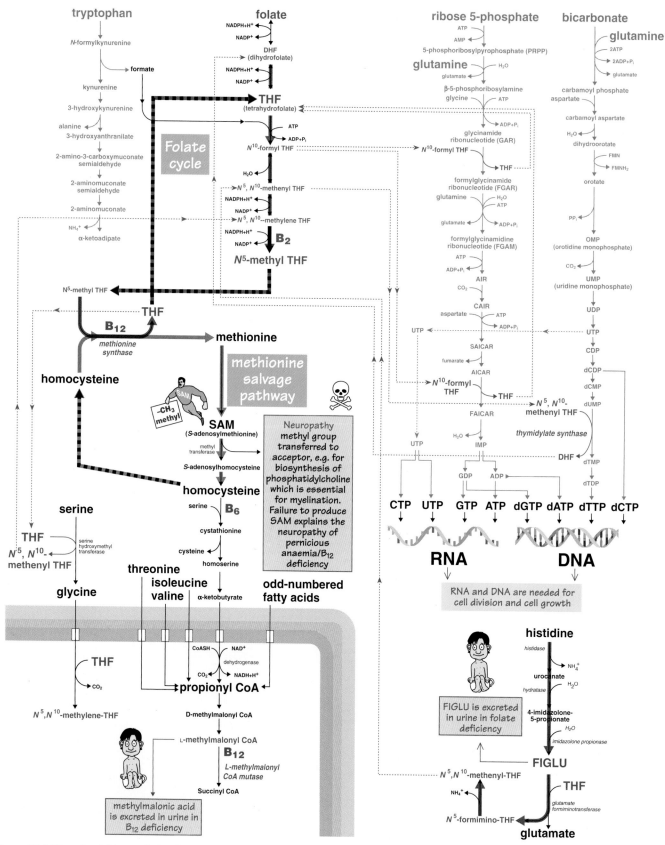

Figure 55.1 The role of folate and vitamin B₁₂ in metabolism.

Vitamin B₁₂

Vitamin B_{12} deficiency is a significant problem, especially in vegetarians and particularly in vegans.

Deficiency is directly related to its two functions, which cause:

1 Secondary folate deficiency resulting in **megaloblastic anaemia** and **neuropathy** (similar to folate deficiency). This is due to the impaired 1-carbon transfer needed for DNA/RNA synthesis and the impaired methyl transfer needed for synthesis of phosphatidylcholine used in myelin formation.

2 Accumulation of methylmalonyl CoA resulting in **neuropathy** (not seen in folate deficiency).

Reference nutrient intake (RNI)

The RNI for vitamin B_{12} is 2 µg/day.

Biochemical functions

Vitamin B_{12} (cobalamin) has two active forms that are involved in two reactions:

1 **Methylcobalamin** is needed for **methionine synthase** (also known as homocysteine methyltransferase) for the **methionine salvage pathway**.

2 **Deoxyadenosylcobalamin** is needed for the **methylmalonyl CoA mutase reaction**.

Diagnostic tests

1 Full blood count and mean cell volume.

2 Measure plasma concentration of cobalamin.

3 Schilling test: radiolabelled vitamin B_{12} is given and urinary excretion is measured. Less than 10% B_{12} excretion suggests deficiency. Pernicious anaemia is confirmed by repeating with intrinsic factor if the excretion of B_{12} is normalised to >10% of the dose.

4 Measure methylmalonic acid in the urine.

Dietary sources

Vegans are vulnerable to vitamin B_{12} deficiency since it is found only in animal products, particularly liver.

Deficiency diseases

1 B_{12} deficiency causes deficient methionine synthase activity, which results in megaloblastic anaemia similar to folate deficiency. In pernicious anaemia the parietal cells of the stomach are destroyed by autoimmune attack and are unable to produce intrinsic factor (50 kDa glycoprotein), which is needed for the absorption of cobalamin in the ileum.

2 B_{12} deficiency causes homocysteinaemia, which is associated with cardiovascular disease.

3 A deficiency of methylmalonyl CoA mutase causes accumulation of methylmalonyl CoA. It is thought that this competes with the normal precursor malonyl CoA for lipid synthesis.

Folate

Serine, tryptophan and histidine donate 1-carbon units to folate metabolites that are used for DNA and RNA synthesis during cell division and growth. NB Vitamin B_{12} is needed for the metabolism and function of folate.

Biochemical functions

Folate is reduced to tetrahydrofolate (THF), which is a carrier of "1-carbon" units:

Formyl	**–CHO**
Methenyl	**–CH=**
Methylene	**–CH₂–**
Methyl	**–CH₃**

These are used for the biosynthesis of the purine and pyrimidine bases in DNA and RNA. Hence THF is vital for cell growth and division.

Diagnostic tests for deficiency

1 Measure plasma/serum folate or red cell folate.

2 Haematology tests for megaloblastic anaemia.

3 Measure **FIGLU** (N-form**imino**glu tamate) after a loading dose of histidine.

Dietary sources

Green leaf vegetables (Latin *folium*, leaf) and also yeast are sources.

Deficiency diseases

1 Folate is needed for cells undergoing rapid division and growth, e.g. haemopoietic tissue in bone marrow. Deficiency causes megaloblastic anaemia.

2 Moderate folate deficiency at the time of conception is associated with neural tube defects, e.g. spina bifida. It is recommended that women who may conceive should take folate supplements of 400 µg daily.

3 Deficiency is associated with hyperhomocysteinaemia, which is a risk factor for cardiovascular disease.

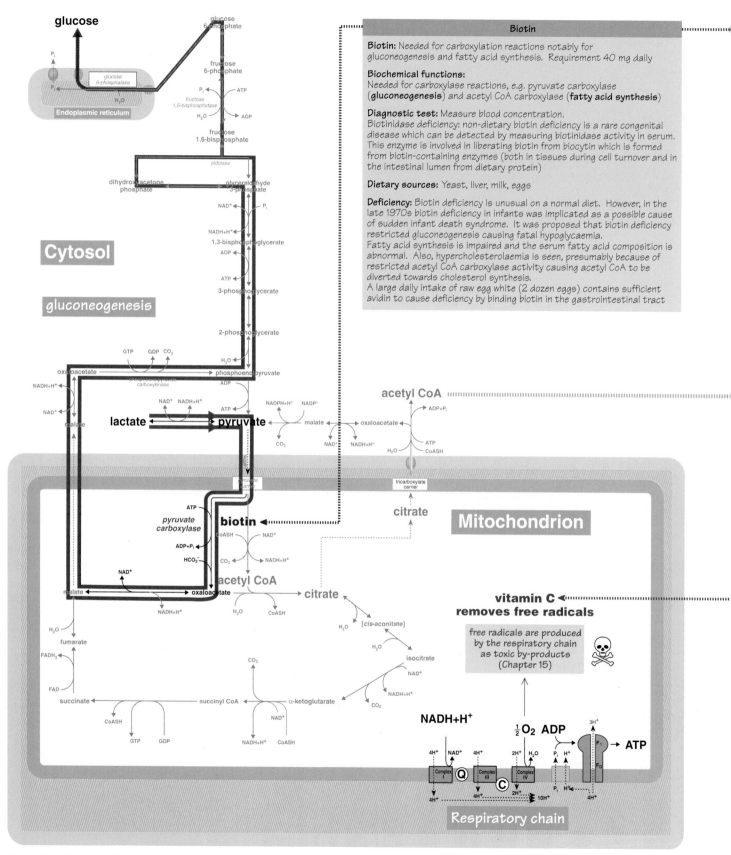

Figure 56.1 The role of biotin and vitamin C in metabolism.

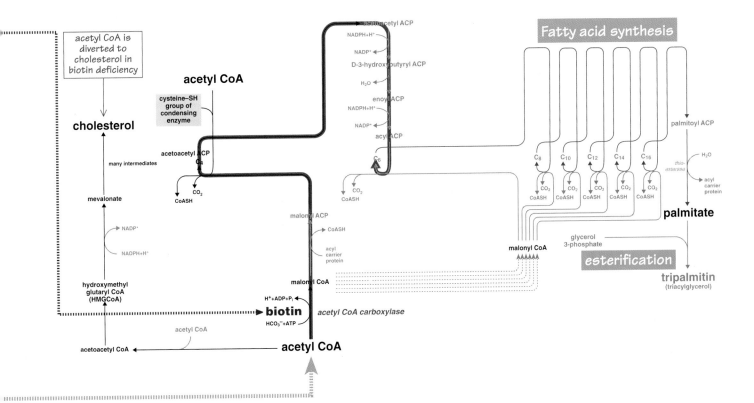

Fatty acid synthesis

acetyl CoA is diverted to cholesterol in biotin deficiency

cholesterol

acetyl CoA

cysteine–SH group of condensing enzyme

acetoacetyl ACP

many intermediates

mevalonate

CO_2
CoASH

NADP⁺ → NADP⁺

NADPH+H⁺

hydroxymethyl glutaryl CoA (HMGCoA)

$H^+ + ADP + P_i$

biotin

$HCO_3^- + ATP$

acetyl CoA carboxylase

acetyl CoA

acetoacetyl CoA

acetyl CoA

acetoacetyl ACP
NADPH+H⁺
NADP⁺
D-3-hydroxybutyryl ACP
H_2O
enoyl ACP
NADPH+H⁺
NADP⁺
acyl ACP

C_6

CO_2
CoASH

malonyl ACP

CoASH

acyl carrier protein

malonyl CoA

malonyl CoA

C_8 C_{10} C_{12} C_{14} C_{16}

CO_2 CO_2 CO_2 CO_2 CO_2
CoASH CoASH CoASH CoASH CoASH

palmitoyl ACP

H_2O
thio-esterase
acyl carrier protein

palmitate

glycerol 3-phosphate

esterification

tripalmitin (triacylglycerol)

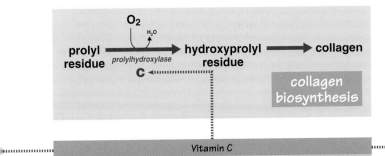

O_2
H_2O

prolyl residue → *prolylhydroxylase* → **hydroxyprolyl residue** → **collagen**

C

collagen biosynthesis

Vitamin C

Vitamin C: Needed for several hydroxylation reactions notably prolyl- and lysylhydroxylase in the formation of collagen (Chapter 8). Also important as a free radical scavenger. Requirements 50 – 60 mg daily

Biochemical functions: Vitamin C (ascorbic acid) is needed for:
(a) Hydroxylation of proline and lysine which is needed for cross-linking in structure of collagen
(b) Functions as a free radical scavenger preventing oxidative damage, e.g. to lipids in cell membranes and LDL (low density lipoproteins); to proteins and to DNA which may cause mutations leading to cancer
(c) Saves vitamin E from oxidative damage
(d) Needed for the biosynthesis of carnitine, noradrenaline. Also needed by the microsomal cytochrome P_{450} enzymes which are involved in the metabolism of drugs and toxic substances

Diagnostic tests: Measure vitamin C in white blood cells ("buffy coat")

Dietary sources: Fresh fruit, particularly citrus fruits, and vegetables

Deficiency: Impaired synthesis of collagen leads to scurvy characterised by bleeding gums, bruising and poor wound-healing.
Vitamin C supplements improve wound-healing and decrease skin-bruising in some types of Ehlers–Danlos syndrome

---

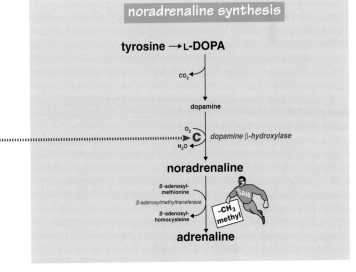

noradrenaline synthesis

tyrosine → L-DOPA

CO_2

dopamine

O_2
C — *dopamine β-hydroxylase*
H_2O

noradrenaline

S-adenosyl-methionine
S-adenosylmethyltransferase
S-adenosyl-homocysteine

–CH_3 methyl

adrenaline

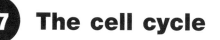

57 The cell cycle

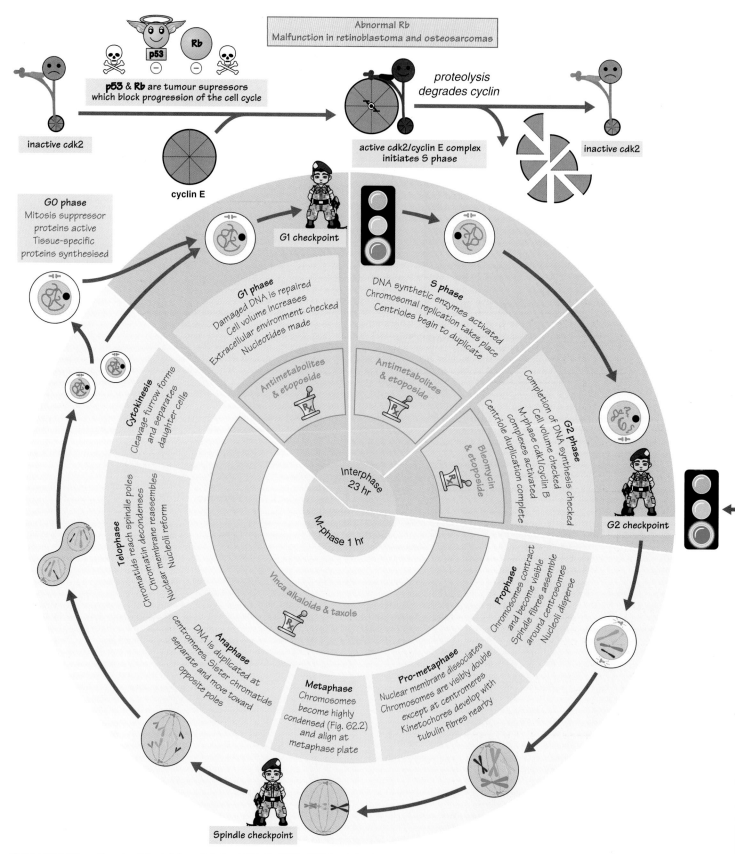

Figure 57.1 The cell cycle. Adapted from Pritchard DJ, Korf BR. (2008) *Medical Genetics at a Glance*, 2nd edn. Blackwell Publishing: Oxford.

Cell function and cell division

At any given moment, most of the cells in the body are performing the function of the tissue or organ of which they are a component. For example they could be involved in metabolic pathways or making hormones and digestive proteins for secretion. However, if they receive a signal from a growth factor they will divide. If cells are damaged by trauma, they can be replaced by division of healthy cells.

The cells of the human body can divide to the extent of many millions per second! During this process the DNA in each cell must be replicated perfectly so each daughter cell is identical to the parent cell. Moreover, the rate of cell division must be balanced with the need for new cells to replace the dying cells. If insufficient cells are produced the tissue will atrophy. If cells are produced at an excessive rate, a tumour is produced. Eukaryotic cells regulate the process of cell division using a sequence of regulatory proteins in the **cell-cycle control system**.

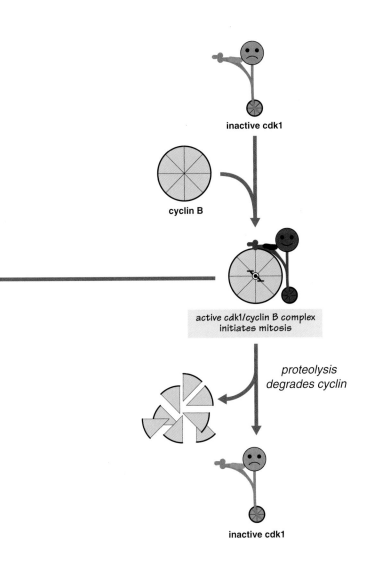

inactive cdk1

cyclin B

active cdk1/cyclin B complex initiates mitosis

proteolysis degrades cyclin

inactive cdk1

Cell-cycle control system

Cell biologists consider the cell cycle to be divided into five phases: **G1, S, G2, M** and **G0**. There are three principal checkpoints at which the cell cycle is stopped if defects are detected: the **G1 checkpoint**, the **G2 checkpoint** and the **spindle checkpoint** during the mitosis phase. The tumour suppressors **p53**, the "**guardian angel protein**", and "**Rb protein**" regulate progression from the G1 phase to the S phase. Mutations of p53 and Rb that fail to suppress progression result in uncontrolled cell division, i.e. tumour development.

1 Gap (or **growth**) **1 phase** (**G1 phase**). This is the principal growth phase during which the cell performs its normal metabolic functions and when nucleotides are made in preparation for DNA synthesis (Chapters 58, 59). At the **G1 checkpoint** checks are made for DNA damage caused by chemicals or ionising radiation (Chapter 65). If damaged DNA is detected, p53 ("guardian angel" tumour suppressor) arrests progression of the cycle. p53 is constitutively expressed in a normal, healthy cell. When DNA damage is detected, p53 stops the cell cycle allowing damaged DNA to be repaired (Chapter 65) before the cell cycle enters the S phase. The tumour suppressor **Rb protein** is also constitutively expressed and in native form inhibits cell cycle progression. For progression to the S phase, Rb becomes hyperphosphorylated which allows the cell cycle to progress. This may be triggered by epidermal growth factor and ultimately culminates in the activation of **c**yclin-**d**ependent **k**inase (cdk)/cyclin complex. As the name suggests, **cdks** are only active when bound to a **cyclin**. During the **S-phase, cyclin E** binds to **cdk2** to form the **active cdk2/cyclin E complex**, which signals the start of the S-phase by triggering **DNA replication** (Chapters 63, 64). The entire genome must be replicated before progression to the Gap 2 phase occurs.

2 Synthetic phase (**S phase**). Synthesis of DNA (replication) occurs and all the chromosomes in the genome are replicated during the S phase.

3 Gap (or **growth**) **2 phase** (**G2 phase**). The cell grows in size, mitochondria replicate, chromosomes condense and proteins (e.g. microtubular proteins) needed for mitosis are made during this phase. The **G2 checkpoint confirms the integrity of DNA and the cell volume**. Providing the check is satisfactory, the mitosis phase is triggered by the active **cdk1/cyclin B complex**.

4 Mitosis phase (**M phase**). The **spindle checkpoint** ensures that all **the chromosomes are correctly aligned** on the spindle fibre prior to cell division.

5 Cytokinesis phase (**C phase**). The **cytokinesis phase** is when the cytoplasm divides, creating two daughter cells.

6 G0 phase. Some types of cell are shunted from the cell cycle into the G0 phase, notably **permanent G0-phase cells**, e.g. red blood cells, neurones and cardiac and skeletal muscle. Permanent cells remain in the G0 phase and must be regenerated from stem cells. Others, e.g. liver cells and lymphocytes, are **stable and enter the G0 phase** where they are quiescent until stimulated to enter the G1 phase by external stimuli. Some cells, e.g. hair follicles and intestinal, epithelial, skin and bone marrow cells, comprise **labile cells** that divide very rapidly. They progress directly to the G1 phase without entering G0.

The **G1 phase, S phase and G2 phase** are collectively known as the **interphase**. The interphase takes typically 23 hours for completion but can be shorter in cancer and gut cells. This is considerably longer than the **mitosis phase** which typically takes only 1 hour.

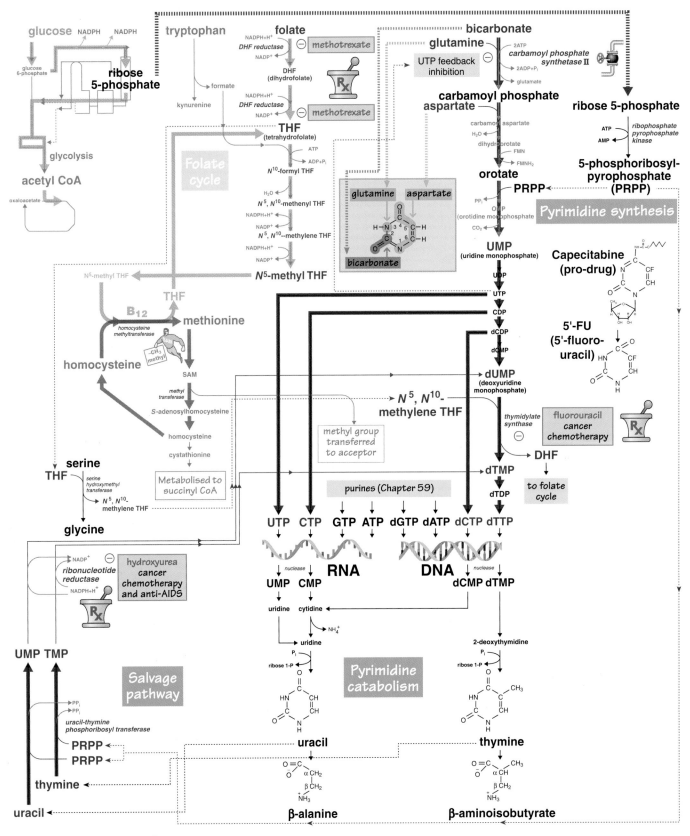

Figure 58.1 Pyrimidine metabolism.

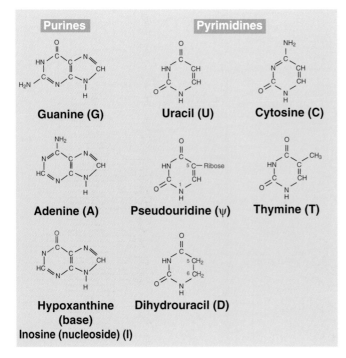

Figure 58.2 Purine and pyrimidine bases.

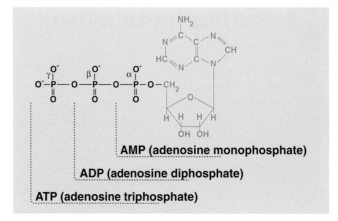

Figure 58.3 Adenosine triphosphate (ATP).

Bases, nucleosides and nucleotides

The **purine bases** are **adenine** (A) and **guanine** (G). The **pyrimidine bases** are **cytosine** (C), **thymine** (T) and **uracil** (U) (Fig. 58.2).

The bases combine with ribose to form their corresponding **nucleosides**: **adenosine, guanosine, cytidine, thymidine** and **uridine**. Alternatively, they combine with **deoxy**ribose to form deoxyadenosine, etc.

The addition of one or more phosphates forms a **nucleotide**, e.g. adenosine (the nucleoside) can form the nucleotides adenosine monophosphate (AMP), adenosine diphosphate (ADP) and **adenosine triphosphate** (ATP) (Fig. 58.3). Alternatively, the corresponding **deoxy**ribonucleotides are formed, e.g. deoxythymidine monophosphate (dTMP).

NB When the bases occur in nucleic acids, adenine, guanine and cytosine are present in both RNA and DNA; uracil is found only in RNA; and thymine is found only in DNA. *Attention: do not confuse "thymine" with vitamin B₁ which is "thiamin".*

Pyrimidines and purines are important for cell growth and division

The pyrimidines and purines have many roles as substrates, coenzymes and signalling molecules and as such play numerous important roles in metabolism. They are major components of DNA and RNA; and are vital for cell growth and division. Not surprisingly, the development and growth of the foetus *in utero* demands a substantial supply of purines and pyrimidines and it is important that the substrates and co-factors needed for their biosynthesis are available to the mother at conception and throughout pregnancy. There is a particular need for **vitamin B₁₂** and **folate** (Chapter 55) and deficiency of these vitamins is associated with birth defects. On the other hand, when an ectopic pregnancy must be terminated, treatment with **methotrexate** (a folate antagonist, see below) has been advocated recently.

Biosynthesis of pyrimidines

The precursors of the pyrimidine ring are **bicarbonate, glutamine** and **aspartate** (Fig. 58.1). The regulatory enzyme is **carbamoylphos-** phate synthetase II (**CPS II**) which is subject to feed-back inhibition by uridine triphosphate (UTP). NB CPS II is different from **CPS I** which provides carbamoyl phosphate for, and is the regulatory enzyme of, the urea cycle (Chapter 44). They differ in that CPS I is a **mitochondrial** enzyme that obtains nitrogen from **ammonia**, while CPS II is **cytosolic** and obtains its nitrogen from the γ-amide of **glutamine**. Another precursor that is needed to methylate **dUMP** to form **dTMP** is N^5,N^{10}-**methylene THF**. dTTP is essential for DNA biosynthesis.

Catabolism of pyrimidines

Cytidine monophosphate (**CMP**) and **dCMP** are deaminated to **uracil** and **dTMP** is degraded to **thymine**. Both uracil and thymine can be recycled to nucleotides by the **salvage pathway**. Alternatively, they can be degraded to **β-alanine** and **β-aminoisobutyrate**, respectively.

Cancer chemotherapy

Cancer cells divide and grow much more rapidly than normal cells and have a great need for DNA and RNA synthesis during the **S** phase (**s**ynthetic) of the "cell cycle" (Fig. 57.1). This provides a strategy for devising anticancer drugs, so folate antagonists, antipyrimidines and antipurines (known as antimetabolites), which inhibit cell proliferation, have been developed.

Folate antagonists

Methotrexate is a close structural analogue of folate and inhibits **dihydrofolate reductase**. This prevents the reduction of folate and dihydrofolate (**DHF**) to tetrahydrofolate (**THF**), which is the precursor of N^5,N^{10}-**methylene THF**. This is essential for dTTP and DNA synthesis. Unfortunately, normal cells are also attacked by methotrexate. Folinic acid (N^5-formyl tetrahydrofolate) is an active form of folate that can be given after the start of methotrexate treatment to rescue normal cells from this drug toxicity.

Antipyrimidines

Anticancer drugs based on pyrimidine analogues containing fluorine (the fluoropyrimidines, e.g. **5-fluorouracil** (5-FU)) have been used successfully to treat cancer. 5-FU acts by inhibiting **thymidylate synthase** thus preventing the methylation of **dUMP** to **dTMP** which is a vital precursor for DNA biosynthesis.

Antipurines

Purine antimetabolites are described in Chapter 59.

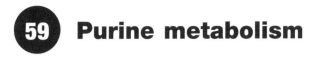

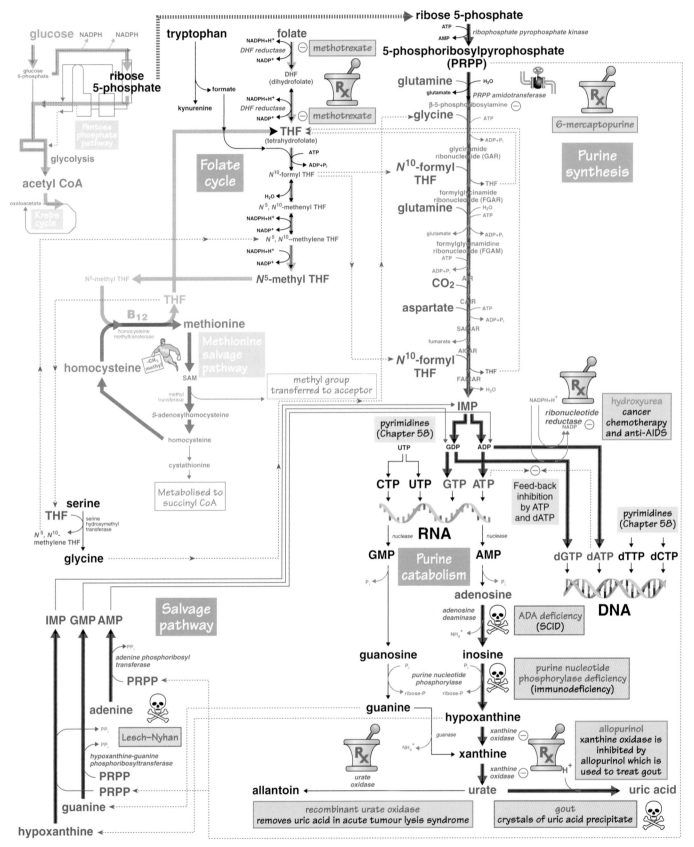

Figure 59.1 Purine metabolism.

Biosynthesis and breakdown of purines

The purine nucleotides GTP and ATP are very important in intermediary metabolism and the regulation of metabolism. Adenine is also a component of cyclic AMP, FAD, NAD$^+$, NADP$^+$ and coenzyme A. Moreover, GTP, ATP and their deoxy derivatives dGTP and dATP are important precursors for the synthesis of RNA and DNA respectively, which are essential for cell growth and division. **Purine biosynthesis** (Fig. 59.1) needs the amino acids **glutamine**, **glycine** and **aspartate**. Also, **tryptophan** is needed to supply formate which reacts with tetrahydrofolate (THF) to produce N^{10}-formyl THF, which donates the **formyl** group to the purine structure. A molecule of CO_2 is also needed.

Purine catabolism produces **urate**, which has the disadvantage of being sparingly soluble in the aqueous environment of blood and has a tendency to precipitate as **uric acid**, with the pathological consequences (gout) described below.

Origin of the atoms in the purine molecule

The origin of the atoms in the purine molecule is shown in Fig. 59.2.

Cancer chemotherapy

Methotrexate, **6-mercaptopurine** and **hydroxyurea** all inhibit the synthesis of purine nucleotides or purine deoxynucleotides. These, respectively, are essential components of RNA and DNA which are vital for cell division and growth. Cancer cells that are dividing and growing rapidly compared with healthy cells, e.g. high-grade lymphomas, are particularly vulnerable to these drugs.

Adenosine deaminase deficiency and severe combined immunodeficiency (SCID)

Adenosine deaminase (ADA) deficiency is a very rare autosomal recessive disease and is responsible for 20–30% of recessively inherited cases of SCID. It causes ATP and dATP to accumulate, which feed-back to inhibit ribonucleotide reductase in thymocytes and peripheral blood B-cells. This in turn restricts the formation of DNA and hence the production of T- and B-cells (SCID). Infants are extremely vulnerable to infection as exemplified by the case in the 1970s of David Vetter who spent his entire life of 12 years protected inside a plastic bubble and is immortalised in the film *The Boy in the Plastic Bubble*. Clinical trials of gene therapy for ADA-SCID are encouraging.

Gout

Gout is commonly associated with rich food and alcohol consumption. Rich food is a source of dietary DNA and RNA, which is broken down to urate. Alcohol causes the accumulation of lactate, which competes with urate for excretion by the kidney. Gout results when the concentration of urate (which is sparingly soluble) in the blood increases to a concentration when it is precipitated as crystals of uric acid. This causes considerable pain, as illustrated in the picture *The Gout* by James Gilray in 1799. The needle-shaped crystals of uric acid can be deposited around joints, especially in the big toe. Crystals can also be deposited in the urinary tract as renal stones or in the skin as tophi, e.g. in the ear lobe. Gout is treated with the xanthine oxidase inhibitor, allopurinol, which restricts the production of uric acid.

Acute tumour lysis syndrome (ATLS)

ATLS is potentially a catastrophic complication of chemotherapy in patients with a high tumour load. It results from cytotoxic damage to large numbers of cancerous cells. The DNA and RNA released are broken down to uric acid, which precipitates in the renal tubules causing acute uric acid nephropathy. Recent evidence suggests that **recombinant urate oxidase**, which converts uric acid to soluble allantoin, is successful in the treatment and prevention of ATLS in patients with haematological malignancies.

Lesch–Nyhan syndrome

Lesch–Nyhan syndrome is a rare, X-linked disorder of **hypoxanthine-guanine phosphoribosyltransferase (HGPRT)** in the purine salvage pathway. This causes severe accumulation of uric acid resulting in gout and renal stones. The condition is characterised by mental retardation and compulsive self-mutilation with biting of the lips, tongue and fingers and head banging. Recombinant urate oxidase has been used in a patient with Lesch-Nyhan syndrome and it reduced plasma urate to normal during the neonatal period. However, allopurinol remains the drug of choice for long-term treatment. (Belén Pérez Dueñas, personal communication.)

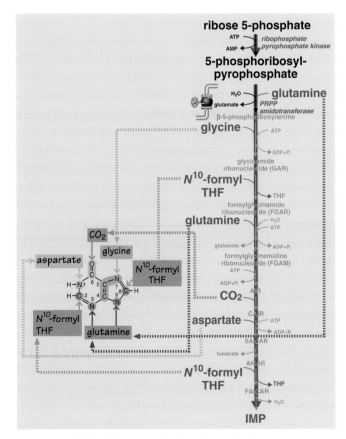

Figure 59.2 Origin of the atoms in the purine molecule.

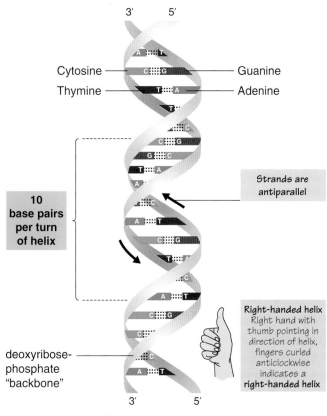

Figure 60.1 Double helix.

The double helix

DNA is a helical structure composed of two strands, the "**double helix**", in which is encoded genetic information. The "backbone" of each strand is composed of a chain of 2′-deoxyribose phosphate molecules joined by phosphodiester bonds (Fig. 60.1). The strands are **antiparallel**, i.e. the strand at the 5′ C end pairs with the 3′ C end of the complementary strand. To the 1′ C of each deoxyribose is joined either a **purine** (**adenine** or **guanine**) or **pyrimidine** (**cytosine** or **thymine**).

Base pairing and "DNA melting" (DNA denaturation)

The two strands of DNA are held together by hydrogen bonds formed between pairs of bases: **adenine pairs with thymine** and **guanine pairs with cytosine** (Fig. 60.2). A single molecule of DNA contains thousands of base pairs. NB **Adenine and thymine** pair with **two** hydrogen bonds (**A=T**), whereas **guanine and cytosine** pair with **three** hydrogen bonds (**G≡C**). This means that the bond between cytosine and guanine is stronger than that between adenine and

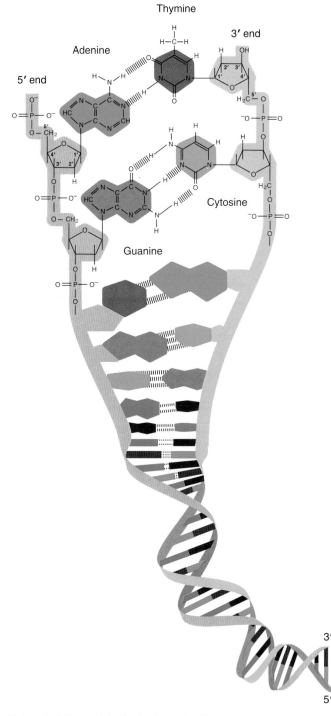

Figure 60.2 Base pairing by hydrogen bonding.

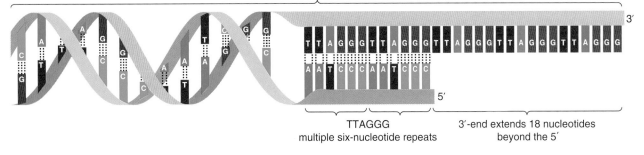

multiple six-nucleotide repeats

TTAGGG

3′-end extends 18 nucleotides
beyond the 5′

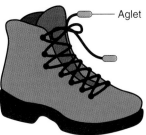

Aglet

Figure 60.3 Telomeres in vertebrates consist of 6-nucleotide repeats: **TTAGGG**.

thymine. Consequently, for DNA with a high proportion of cytosine and guanine, a higher melting temperature is needed to separate the double-stranded DNA into single strands.

Telomeres and telomerase

The Nobel Prize in Physiology or Medicine 2009 was awarded for the discovery of "*How chromosomes are protected by telomeres and telomerase*". **Telomeres** are the caps at both ends of the chromosomal DNA helix and have been likened to **aglets**, which stop shoe laces fraying (Fig. 60.3). In vertebrates, telomeres are repeats of the sequence **TTAGGG** which attracts proteins forming a protective cap at the fragile end of the DNA strand. Telomeres are made by **telomerase**, which contains both protein and RNA. The RNA provides the template for synthesising telomere DNA. Telomerase is reduced in ageing cells and cancer cells resulting in chromosomal instability and further cellular damage.

The "central dogma" of molecular biology

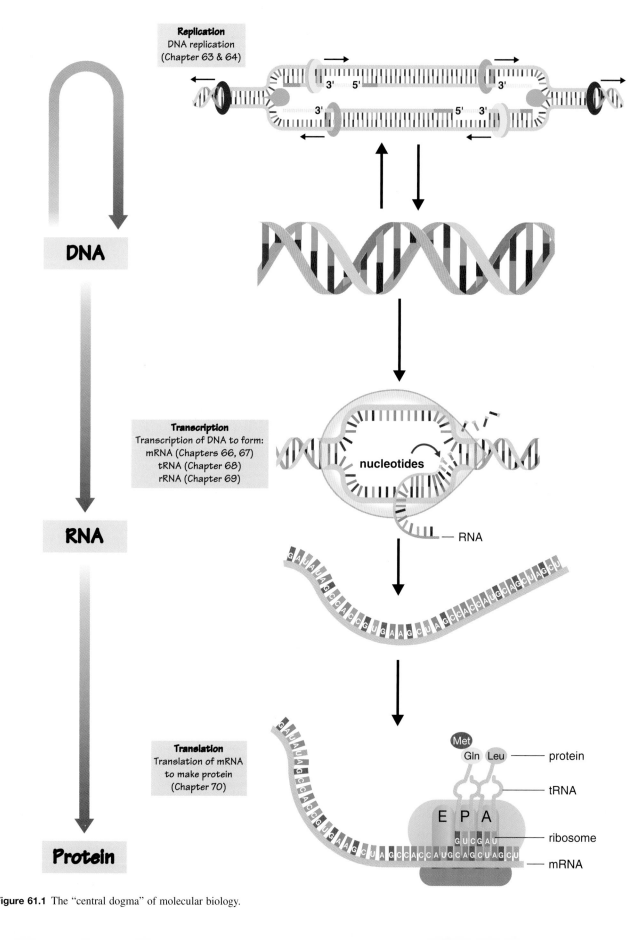

Figure 61.1 The "central dogma" of molecular biology.

Central dogma

The "central dogma" formulated by Francis Crick in 1958 states that the flow of genetic information is from DNA to RNA to protein as follows:

DNA → RNA → protein

The details are summarised in Fig. 61.1. There are three processes by which this flow is achieved:

1 Replication. Replication is the process by which a DNA double helix makes an identical copy of itself using the parent strands as templates or patterns (Chapters 63 and 64).

2 Transcription. Transcription is the process by which the genetic code stored in the DNA is transcribed to make RNA. This can be messenger RNA (mRNA; Chapters 66 and 67), transfer RNA (tRNA; Chapter 68) or ribosomal RNA (rRNA; Chapter 69). mRNA contains the coded instructions for the amino acid sequence in proteins. It should be noted that in eukaryotes only 2% or less of the DNA is informational (i.e. genes). The rest has structural, regulatory and protective functions, or may be just "junk".

3 Translation. Translation is the process by which the instructions encoded in mRNA are used, in conjunction with tRNA and ribosomes, to determine the sequence of amino acids during protein synthesis (Chapter 70).

Exceptions to the central dogma

Inevitably, in the decades since Crick formulated the central dogma it has been challenged, notably by the discovery of **RNA viruses** and **prions**.

RNA viruses contain RNA as their genetic material. They can be single- or double-stranded RNA viruses, e.g. influenza virus, and they replicate using a special viral RNA polymerase. The retroviruses, e.g. human immunodeficiency virus (HIV), replicate inside their host cell using **reverse transcriptase**, producing DNA that becomes integrated within the host genome.

A **prion** (**pr**oteinaceous **in**fectious + **on**) is a microscopic particle of protein that causes neurological diseases such as Creutzfeldt–Jakob disease (CJD) (Chapter 7). Prions multiply by catalysing the misfolding of normal cellular prion proteins (PrP^C) into malignant prion forms (e.g. the scrapie prion PrP^{SC}) without the participation of DNA and RNA.

Genetic code

The genetic code is based on triplet codons composed of three bases. Each triplet corresponds to a specific amino acid (Table 61.1). The mRNA codon **AUG** signals the start of a polypeptide reading frame in which the triplet codons determine the sequence of amino acids. The mRNA stop codons are: UAA, UGA, UAG.

Features of the genetic code

1 Unambiguous. Each codon encodes only one amino acid. An exception is in **prokaryotes. The translation start signal is *N*-formylmethionine (fMet)**. This enters the ribosome at the P-site (Chapter 70) where it is subject to "wobble" on the **first** position of the codon (Chapter 68). Thus, although **AUG** is the major start codon, a significant number of genes start with **GUG, UUG or CUG**. In both **pro- and eukaryotes, AUG codes for all methionine** molecules within the subsequent reading frames.

2 Degenerate. Amino acids are specified by more than one codon, for example arginine, serine and leucine have six codons. **Leucine** is coded by UUA, UUG, CUU, CUC, CUA and CUG. The exceptions are **methionine** and **tryptophan** which each have a single codon, AUG and UGG, respectively.

3 Unpunctuated and non-overlapping. The code is read from a fixed starting point (AUG) with the triplet codon as a reading frame. The code is a continuous sequence of bases, i.e. there are no punctuation gaps between codons. Moreover, codons do not overlap.

4 Universal. Amazingly, the genetic code has been conserved throughout evolution and is the same in nearly all living organisms from microscopic bacteria to the colossal blue whales. There are a few exceptions, notably mitochondrial DNA.

Table 61.1 The genetic code is composed of triplets of three bases. For example, UUU codes for the amino acid phenylalanine and UCU codes for serine.

Base in 1st position	Base in 2nd position				Base in 3rd 'wobble' position
	U	**C**	**A**	**G**	
U	Phe	Ser	Tyr	Cys	U
	Phe	Ser	Tyr	Cys	C
	Leu	Ser	STOP!	STOP!	A
	Leu	Ser	STOP!	Trp	G
C	Leu	Pro	His	Arg	U
	Leu	Pro	His	Arg	C
	Leu	Pro	Gln	Arg	A
	Leu	Pro	Gln	Arg	G
A	Ile	Thr	Asn	Ser	U
	Ile	Thr	Asn	Ser	C
	Ile	Thr	Lys	Arg	A
	Met or START	Thr	Lys	Arg	G
G	Val	Ala	Asp	Gly	U
	Val	Ala	Asp	Gly	C
	Val	Ala	Glu	Gly	A
	Val	Ala	Glu	Gly	G
	Amino acids				

Table 61.2 The genetic code. By convention, the genetic code is based on the sequence of bases, read from 5′ to 3′ in mRNA. For example, CUA specifies the amino acid leucine. Note that in DNA, the corresponding "coding strand" is CTA (in RNA U replaces T). The complementary "template strand" of DNA is GAT. This corresponds to the base pairing in the DNA helix (Fig. 60.1), i.e. C≡G and A=T.

DNA	Coding strand	5′	ATG	AAG	CTA	GCT	3′
	Template strand	3′	TAC	TTC	GAT	CGA	5′
mRNA		5′	AUG	AAG	CUA	GCU	3′
Protein amino acids	N		Met or START!	Lys	Leu	Ala	C

62 Organisation of DNA in chromosomes

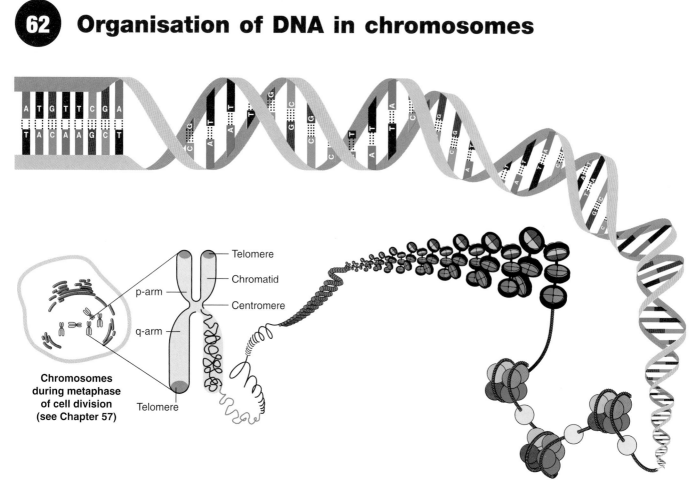

Figure 62.1 DNA combines with protein to form chromatin, which enables packing within the nucleus.

Organisation of DNA in eukaryotes

The total length of the main nuclear DNA is subdivided into 23 pairs of chromosomes in humans. The **total length of DNA is 2 m** so the **average length of DNA per individual chromosome** is approximately **4 cm**. DNA is approximately 2 nm wide. If scaled in proportion to knitting wool 2 mm wide, the total length would be 2000 km or 1250 miles. All this DNA must be organised and structured within the cell nucleus and must be: (i) capable of replication during cell division, and (ii) capable of transcription to produce RNA. Imagine if the chromosomal DNA was like 23 balls of wool: obviously there is the potential for chaos and a desperate tangle (Fig. 62.3). The organisation of DNA is summarised in Figures 62.1 and 62.2.

Mitochondrial DNA (mtDNA)

A small proportion of human DNA is mtDNA contained within mitochondria that is involved in making some of the mitochondrial proteins. Mitochondria are thought to be the ghosts of ancient bacterial cells that, millions of years ago, established a symbiotic relationship (endosymbiosis) with what are now known as eukaryotic cells. As would be expected, mtDNA has a circular, double-stranded structure similar to prokaryotic DNA (Fig. 63.4). mtDNA is inherited maternally. This is because the sperm cells do not contribute mitochondria to the egg during fertilisation.

Organisation of DNA in prokaryotes
Chromosomal DNA

In prokaryotes, the chromosomal DNA is a circular molecule of

double-stranded DNA associated with proteins. Its size varies from 160,000 to 12,000,000 base pairs (Fig. 63.4).

Plasmid DNA

Plasmids are small circles of DNA containing approximately 1000–200,000 base pairs. These are involved in the rapid transfer of genes, e.g. antibiotic resistance, between bacterial species.

Organisation of DNA in viruses

Viruses contain either DNA or RNA. In DNA viruses, the DNA is **double-stranded (dsDNA)** except, for example, in the parvovirus which is a very small structure, approximately 25 nm in diameter, and made of **single-stranded DNA (ssDNA)** (Latin *parvus*, small). Most DNA viruses are linear molecules except for papilloma, polyoma and hepadnaviruses (e.g. hepatitis B) which are circular.

Chromatin, euchromatin and heterochromatin

1 Chromatin is composed of DNA plus packing and regulatory proteins.
2 Euchromatin is a less condensed, relaxed form of chromatin that participates in transcription.
3 Heterochromatin is a highly condensed, tight form of chromatin that is unable to participate in transcription.
In different cell types, different batteries of genes are working. This is reflected in the condensed/decondensed state of chromatin. During cell division, all the nuclear DNA is highly condensed into the

DNA double helix

2 nm diameter: packing ratio 1

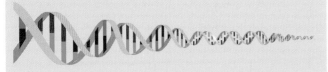

Solenoid (Greek *solen,* pipe) or 30 nm chromatin fibre

30 nm diameter: packing ratio 50:1

Interphase

The nucleosomes coil to make a **30 nm chromatin fibre** (six nucleosomes per turn)

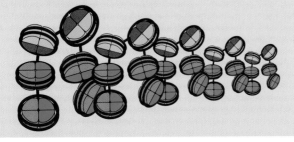

Loop domains

250 nm: packing ratio 250:1

The chromatin fibres form a series of loops which are fixed to a scaffold matrix (50 loops per turn). The scaffold matrix is made of a **"non-histone chromosomal protein"**

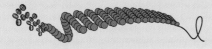

Heterochromatin

840 nm: packing ratio 5000:1

A highly condensed form of chromatin organised as loops in rosette-like structures. The loops are coiled to form the chromosome (18 loops per turn)

Nucleosomes: the "beads on a string" form of chromatin

11 nm diameter: packing ratio 10:1

DNA combines with **histones** to form **chromatin**. Histones are proteins rich in the basic amino acids lysine and arginine and so have a **positive charge**. Two copies of each of the four histones, **H2A**, **H2B**, **H3** and **H4**, combine as an **octamer** to form the "bead". The "string" is DNA with a **negative charge** due to the phosphate groups. The DNA wraps twice around the octamer to form the **nucleosome**. A fifth histone, H1 known as the **"linker histone"**, organises the architectural structure of the nucleosome

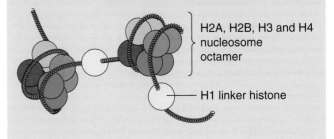

H2A, H2B, H3 and H4 nucleosome octamer

H1 linker histone

Metaphase chromosome

840 nm diameter: packing ratio 5000:1

The chromosome is composed of two chromatids joined at the centromere

p-arm: *petit*, French for small. The short arm

q-arm: Long arm (because **q** follows **p** in the alphabet)

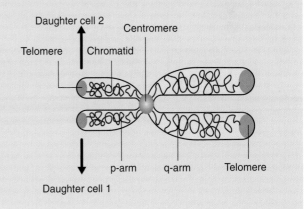

Daughter cell 2

Centromere

Telomere

Chromatid

p-arm q-arm Telomere

Daughter cell 1

Figure 62.2 DNA is tightly packed enabling it to fit within the cell nucleus.

metaphasic chromosome (Fig. 62.2). After cell division, the nuclear DNA decondenses and the genes recommence transcription/translation. During development, **DNA methylation**, which reults in inactivation of gene expression, may modify gene expression so the daughter cells differ in function from the mother cell.

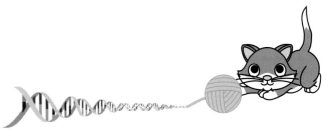

Figure 62.3 The long coil of DNA could become a chaotic tangle!

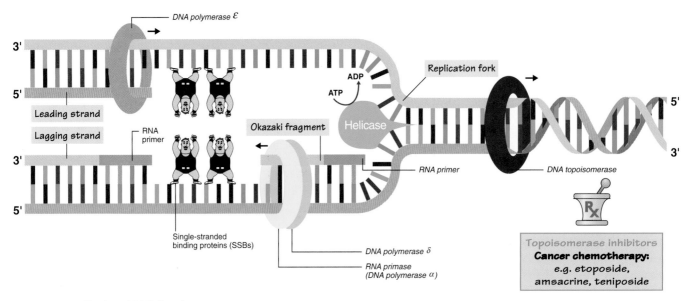

Figure 63.1 Replication of DNA in eukaryotes.

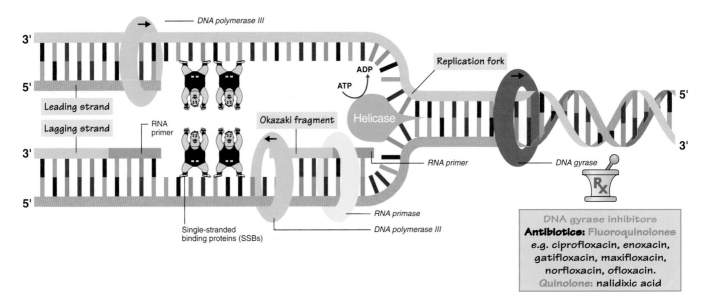

Figure 63.2 Replication of DNA in prokaryotes.

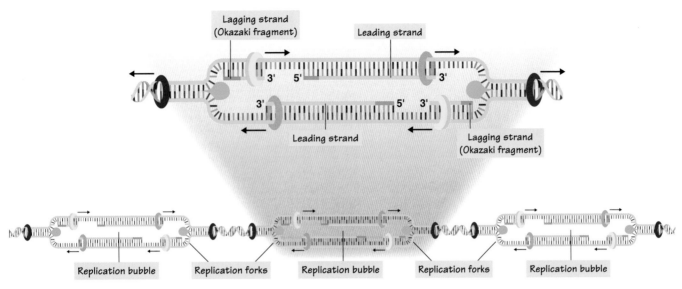

Figure 63.3 Multiple replication bubbles in eukaryotes.

DNA replication occurs during cell growth

During cell growth, DNA (the genetic material) must be copied with high fidelity for inheritance by the daughter cells. This process is called **DNA replication**. It involves several types of DNA polymerase that attach the **5′-phosphate** of the deoxyribonucleotides, dATP, dGTP, dTTP and dCTP, to the **3′-hydroxyl** group of the growing DNA strand.

Replication of DNA in both **eukaryotes** and **prokaryotes** has much in common. However, there are important differences in detail. These differences are emphasised below and in Figs 63.1 to 63.4. In Chapter 71 the details of prokaryotic and eukaryotic DNA replication are compared and contrasted in tabular form.

Origin of replication

Eukaryotes tend to have much more DNA than prokaryotes. Therefore, to speed the process of replication it occurs in **multiple replication bubbles** (Fig. 63.3). Within each bubble, DNA replication occurs at two **replication forks**. However, in **prokaryotes** there is only a **single replication bubble** (Fig. 63.4). In both prokaryotes and eukaryotes, the consensus sequence at an "**origin of replication**" varies but all have a **high content of A and T**, which facilitates separation of the strands. Remember that **A=T** bonds (two hydrogen bonds) are more easily separated than **C≡G** bonds (three hydrogen bonds).

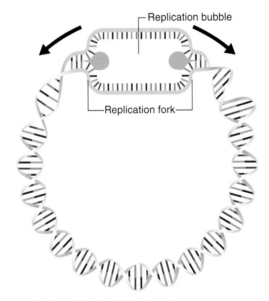

Figure 63.4 Single replication bubble in prokaryotes.

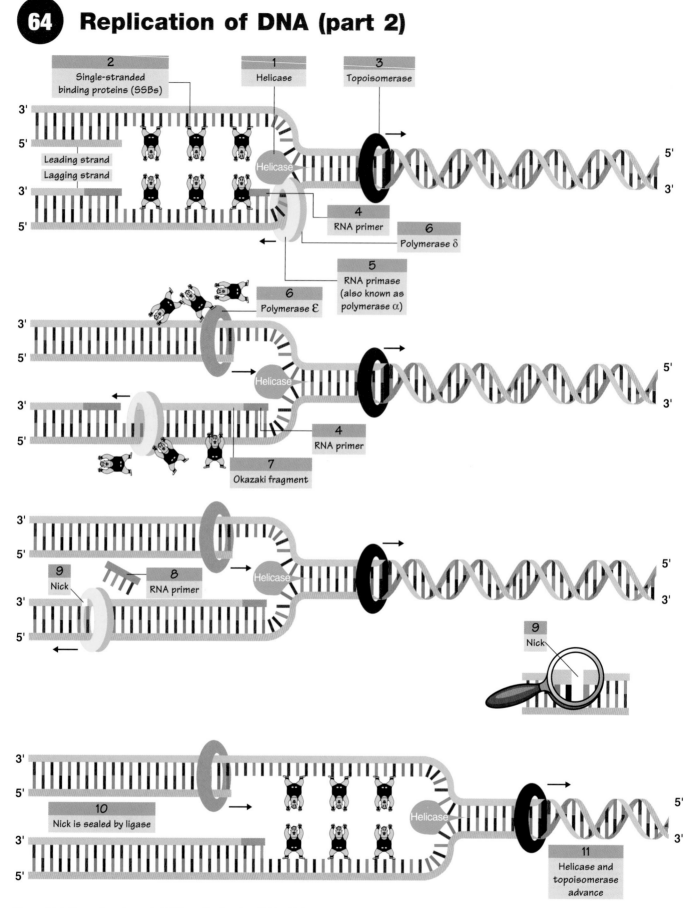

Figure 64.1 Stages in eukaryotic DNA replication (see Table 64.1 *opposite*).

Replication of the DNA double helix

DNA replication is **semiconservative**. The double strand separates progressively into two single strands, each forming a template for replication. Each new DNA formed contains one strand of the original DNA and one strand of new DNA. During replication the **base-pairing rules** are observed. Wherever there is an **A** (or **T**) in the template strand, a **T** (or **A**) is placed. Similarly, wherever there is a **G** (or **C**), a **C** (or **G**) is placed. Thus, the two daughter DNA helices are identical to the mother helix. The following processes occur in replication:

• **"Unzipping" DNA**. The two strands separate, exposing two complementary copies of single-stranded DNA. They are forced apart by **DNA helicase** at the **replication fork**.

• **Single-stranded binding proteins** (SSBs) prevent the strands from rejoining and strongly stimulate helicase activity.

• **Topoisomerase in eukaryotes (gyrase in prokaryotes) prevents supercoiling**. Unwinding the double helix causes positive supercoiling ahead of the advancing helicase. The stresses of supercoiling are relieved by **topoisomerase/gyrase**, which break both DNA strands, pass a double helix through the gap and then rejoin them.

• **Histones**. During replication the histones are displaced and they rejoin later to repackage the new double helix.

• **DNA polymerases**. Several types of DNA polymerase make DNA by adding the deoxyribonucleotides dATP, dGTP, dTTP and dCTP to the free **3′-OH** at the end of the DNA. These enzymes can only read the **template DNA** in the direction **3′ → 5′. In eukaryotes, the identity of the polymerases is not fully understood** (Table 71.1). The currently favoured model (see Fig. 64.1) suggests that **polymerase ε** is the primary "leading strand" replicase. This grows **continuously towards the fork in the direction 3′ → 5′. Polymerases α** and **δ** cooperate to synthesise the **lagging strand.**[*]

• **Lagging strand. Problem!** Remember, DNA polymerase reads the template DNA in the direction **3′ → 5′**; this means **away** from the fork. In other words, it is growing the wrong way! The solution is that **DNA grows discontinuously away from the fork** producing a series of **Okazaki fragments**, as follows. A **complex of DNA polymerase α and polymerase δ** is involved. First, **DNA polymerase α** (an **RNA primase**) makes an **RNA primer**. Then, **polymerase δ** forms a short length of DNA (an **Okazaki fragment**) stopping to leave a **nick** adjacent to the previous RNA primer. Next, this RNA primer is removed, the gap is filled in and the loose ends are joined by **DNA ligase**.

[*] Kunkel TA, Burgers PM. (2008) Dividing the workload at a eukaryotic replication fork. *Trends Cell Biol* **18**(11), 521–7. Also Juhani Syvoaja, personal communication.

Table 64.1 DNA replication in eukaryotes. Numbers refer to Figure 64.1 *opposite*.

1	**DNA helicase** and **replication fork**	DNA **helicase** unwinds the DNA double helix at the Y-shaped "**replication fork**"
2	**Single-stranded binding proteins**	Keep the single strands apart at the replication fork preventing them from rejoining (re-annealing)
3	**Super-coiling caused by helicase**	**Topoisomerase** cuts and rejoins the DNA helix to relieve positive supercoiling
4	**RNA primer**	**Leading** strand needs only **one** RNA primer. **Lagging strand** needs an RNA primer for **each Okazaki fragment**
5	**RNA primase**	**DNA polymerase α** (also known as RNA primase) associates with DNA **polymerase δ** forming a complex. **Primase** makes the **RNA primer** to which DNA is added by DNA polymerase δ
6	**DNA polymerases**	**Polymerase δ:** Makes DNA on the lagging strand (Okazaki fragments) **Polymerase ε:** Makes DNA on the leading strand
7	**Okazaki fragments**	Approximately 100–200 deoxynucleotides
8	**Removal of RNA primer leaves a "gap" which is filled with DNA**	**Single primer from the leading strand; multiple primers from lagging strand** removed by **RNase H** (RNase **H**: acts on a **Hybrid** of RNA and DNA). **Polymerase δ** makes DNA to fill the gap vacated by the RNA primer
9,10	**DNA ligase seals the "nick"**	A **nick** remains at the 3′-hydroxy end of the Okazaki fragment. DNA ligase joins this 3′-hydroxy to the adjacent free 5′-phosphate group forming a phosphodiester bond
11	**Helicase and topoisomerase**	Helicase and topoisomerase advance along the DNA chain

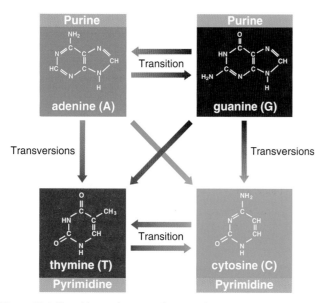

Figure 65.1 Transition and transversion mutations.

DNA mutations differ from DNA damage

Although replication is very accurate, each day in a single cell, up to 10,000 bases are damaged or erroneously inserted into DNA! *NB DNA damage is different from DNA mutation.*

DNA mutations are **inheritable changes** to the sequence of bases. Mutations, comprising matching base pairs, cannot be detected and so therefore cannot be repaired. Mutations can be benign, particularly if they occur in non-coding DNA. However, sometimes they cause the production of functionally abnormal proteins resulting in disease.

Point mutations are changes to a **single base**. They are classified as either "**transition mutations**" or "**transversion mutations**" (Fig. 65.1). **Transitions** are an interchange of **a purine for a purine** or **a pyrimidine for a pyrimidine. Transversions** are an interchange of **a purine for a pyrimidine.**

DNA damage

DNA damage includes **DNA polymerase errors** (deletion or insertion of bases), **strand breaks** caused by X-rays, and **cross-linking** (e.g. psoralen) between duplex strands that prevents strand separation, e.g. thymine cross-linking across the duplex.

DNA damage occurs when the DNA structure is distorted and physically abnormal. Normal oxidative metabolism, ionising radiation and ultraviolet light produce **reactive oxygen species (ROS)** (Chapter 15). ROS cause damage by oxidising guanine to 8-oxo-7,8-dihydroguanine (8-oxoguanine), and uracil to 5-hydroxymethyldeoxyuracil. ROS also damage DNA by causing strand breaks. Ultraviolet light directly damages DNA by causing adjacent pyrimidines to dimerise covalently (Fig. 65.2). Dimerisation of adjacent thymine molecules creates an abnormality that distorts the DNA helix.

Spontaneous deamination of bases

A common cause of DNA damage results from spontaneous deamination of bases, for example spontaneous deamination of **cytosine** forms **uracil** (Fig. 65.2). Remember **uracil** is found in **RNA** and is not normally present in DNA. In RNA, **uracil pairs with adenine**. Also, remember **cytosine pairs with guanine** so if the cytosine is deaminated to uracil an incompatible pairing of the uracil with guanine results that distorts the DNA helix. This type of "single base damage" is repaired by the **base excision repair** process.

DNA repair
Base excision repair process

Base excision is used to correct defects involving a **single base**. Figure 65.2 shows how the erroneous base **uracil** (derived from cytosine) is cleaved from the 1′ C of deoxyribose by **DNA glycosylase** to leave an "**AP site**" (for structure of DNA, see Fig. 60.2). An AP site is a site without either a purine or a pyrimidine – described as "**apurinic**" or "**apyrimidinic**". Alternatively, it is known as an "**abasic site**". Then **AP endonuclease** cleaves the 5′ C bond. This is followed by **deoxyribose phosphate lyase** that removes **deoxyribose phosphate** by cleaving the 3′ C bond. Finally, the gap is filled by **DNA polymerase** and the nick is sealed by **DNA ligase**.

Nucleotide excision repair process

Nucleotide excision is used to repair DNA damage affecting more than a single base or bulky damage, e.g. distortion to the double helix caused by Benzo[*a*]pyrene or aflatoxin. The process involves **specialised endonucleases**. This removes an **oligonucleotide** that includes the damaged bases. In the example shown in Fig. 65.2, **UV-specific endonuclease** removes damage resulting from dimerisation of two thymine bases. Finally, the gap is filled by **DNA polymerase** and the nick is sealed by **DNA ligase**.

Xeroderma pigmentosa is a rare, autosomal recessive disease caused by a defective UV-specific endonuclease. Patients with mutations are unable to repair DNA damage caused by sunlight and have been described as "children of the night".

Mismatched base repair process

Mismatched bases produced during DNA replication are those not conforming to C≡G or A=T base pairing. They are identified and corrected in the new strand by the "**mismatch-repair enzyme complex**". The mismatched nucleotides are identified and excised, and the gap filled by DNA polymerase. Mutations in this complex result in failure to correct mismatched base pairs and cause **hereditary non-polyposis colorectal cancer (HNPCC)**.

Double-strand damage and chromosome breakage

Ionising radiation can cause double-strand damage. If this happens, then the repair process may not be completely accurate, resulting in a mutation in the DNA and possibly cellular malfunction, e.g. skin cancer.

Some cancers have irreparable chromosome breakage in the later stages of tumour development.

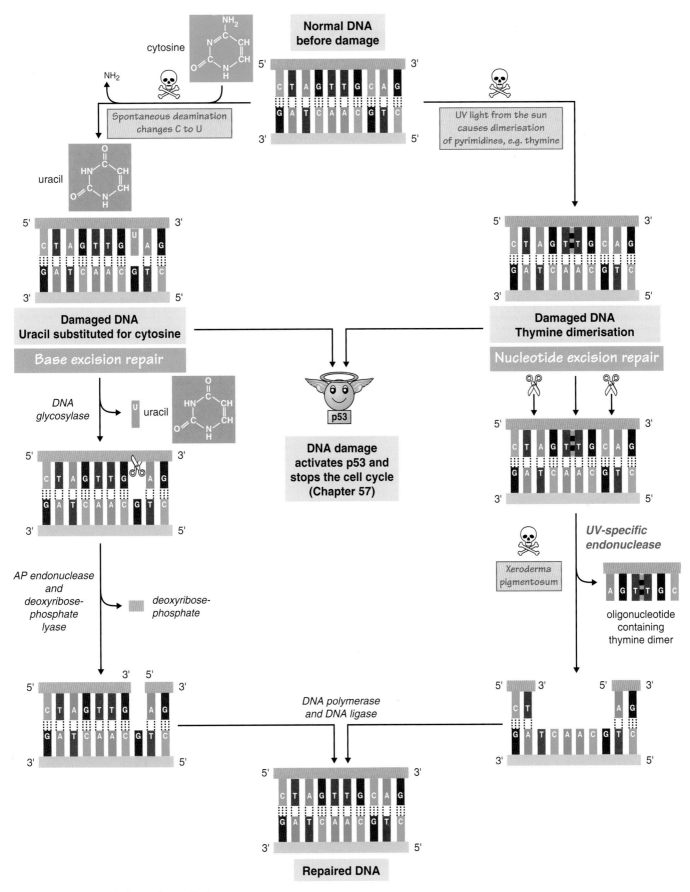

Figure 65.2 Damaged DNA can be repaired.

Transcription of DNA to make messenger RNA (part 1)

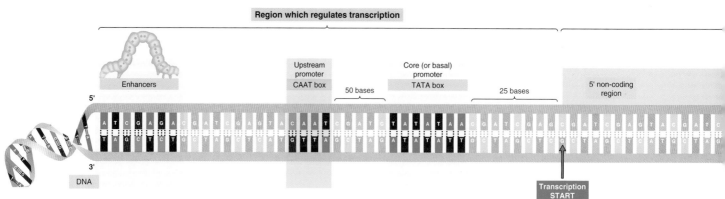

Figure 66.1 Transcription of DNA in eukaryotes to make mRNA.

Messenger RNA in eukaryotes

RNA polymerase II makes mRNA in the nucleus from the nucleotides ATP, GTP, CTP and UTP (not TTP) using the template strand of DNA (Fig. 66.2). Figure 66.1 shows the process of transcription.

1 Initiation of transcription. Transcription factors (e.g. SREBP; Chapter 31) bind to the **promoter regions** (**TATA** (Hogness) box and **CAAT** box) of the gene and recruit **RNA polymerase II**. *(These are consensus sequences, i.e. they represent the bases most frequently found in these positions, although many such sequences contain variations from this pattern.)* This starts the process of transcription. The TATA and CAAT boxes are rich in **A=T** paired bases, i.e. with relatively weak hydrogen bonding, a property that facilitates opening of the DNA double helix to form a "**transcription bubble**" (Fig. 66.2). Now polymerase II attracts the trinucleotides **ATP**, **GTP**, **UTP** and **CTP** to the template strand of DNA according to the base-pairing rules, and polymerisation to form RNA begins. At some distance upstream from the TATA box is the **enhancer** region that also binds transcription factors. This loops towards the RNA polymerase and enhances the rate of transcription.

2 Elongation. Polymerase II moves along the DNA strand with transcription of the DNA occurring in the **transcription bubble** forming the primary transcript **pre-mRNA**.

3 Silencers. Transcription is repressed by **inhibitory regulators** that bind to the **silencer** region of the gene. Silencers (not shown in Fig. 66.1) might be situated some distance from the gene they regulate. However, they can loop over to interact with RNA polymerase and inhibit transcription.

4 Termination. Termination of transcription in eukaryotes is poorly understood.

5 Pre-messenger RNA (pre-mRNA). The first product of DNA transcription by **RNA polymerase II** is **pre-mRNA**. It has a **cap**, a **tail**, non-coding **introns** and coding **exons** and must be modified extensively inside the nucleus before it is exported to the cytosol as mature mRNA.

6 Guanosine cap. GTP and SAM make methylated guanosine triphosphate (**methylated GTP**) to form the **7-methylguanosine cap** (**7-MG cap**) that protects the 5′ end.

7 Poly-A tail. After transcription, and without a DNA template, **poly-A polymerase** adds 100–250 molecules of ATP to the 3′ end of pre-mRNA, forming the "**poly-A tail**". Its formation is signalled by the **polyadenylation sequence** "AAUAAA" at the 3′ end. The poly-A tail facilitates export of mature mRNA from the nucleus and delays its degradation. The longer the poly-A tail, the longer the mRNA half-life and vice versa. Degradation of mRNA controls the steady-state of gene expression. Those mRNA species with a short half-life (<1 hour) are

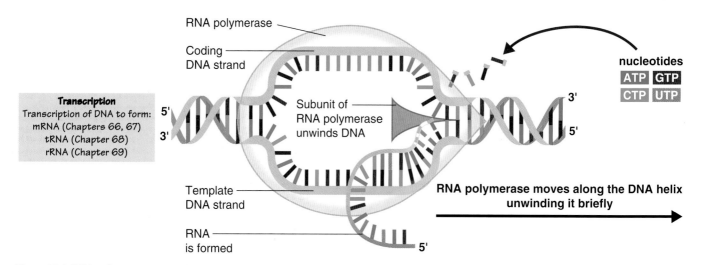

Figure 66.2 RNA polymerase moves along the DNA helix and transcribes the template DNA strand in a "transcription bubble".

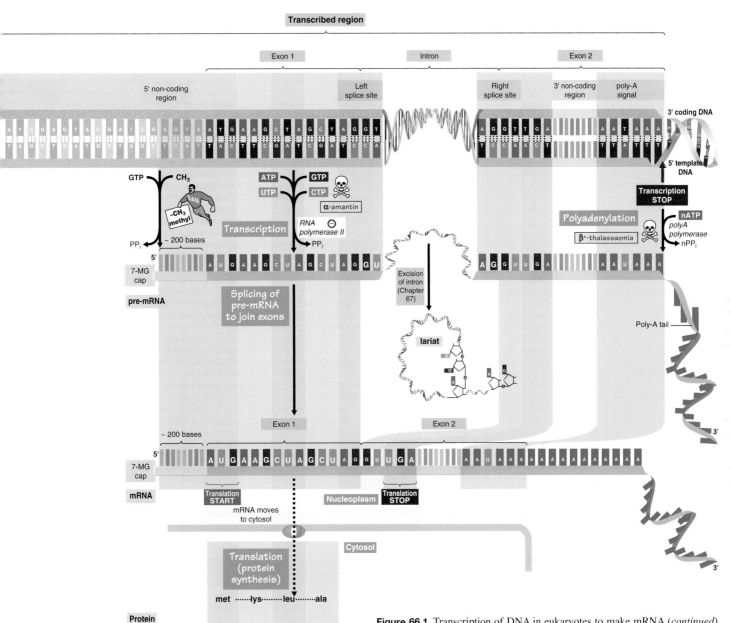

Figure 66.1 Transcription of DNA in eukaryotes to make mRNA (*continued*).

associated with genes whose products have regulatory functions, e.g. controlling the cell cycle. Species of mRNA with a long half-life (5–24 hours) are expressed by "house-keeping" genes, e.g. those associated with metabolism and protein synthesis.

8 Processing of pre-mRNA. The excision of introns, and the splicing of exons, is described in Chapter 67.

B⁺-thalassaemia

Caused, in some patients, by a point mutation at the "**poly-A signal site**" where **AATAAA** becomes **AACAAA**. Homozygous patients have impaired ability to produce β-chain mRNA for the synthesis of the β-globin component of haemoglobin. This results in severe anaemia.

Death cap mushrooms

RNA polymerase II is inhibited by **α-amanitin**, the toxin of the death cap mushroom (*Amanita phalloides*), which, if eaten, can be fatal.

Eukaryotes

In eukaryotes, messenger RNA (mRNA) is made by **RNA polymerase II**, transfer RNA is made by **RNA polymerase III** (Chapter 68) and ribosomal RNA is made by both **RNA polymerase I** and **RNA polymerase III** (for 5S RNA) (Chapter 69).

Prokaryotes

Although there are many similarities in prokaryote and eukaryote transcription, the principal differences are summarised in Table 71.2.

Transcription of DNA to make messenger RNA (part 2)

67

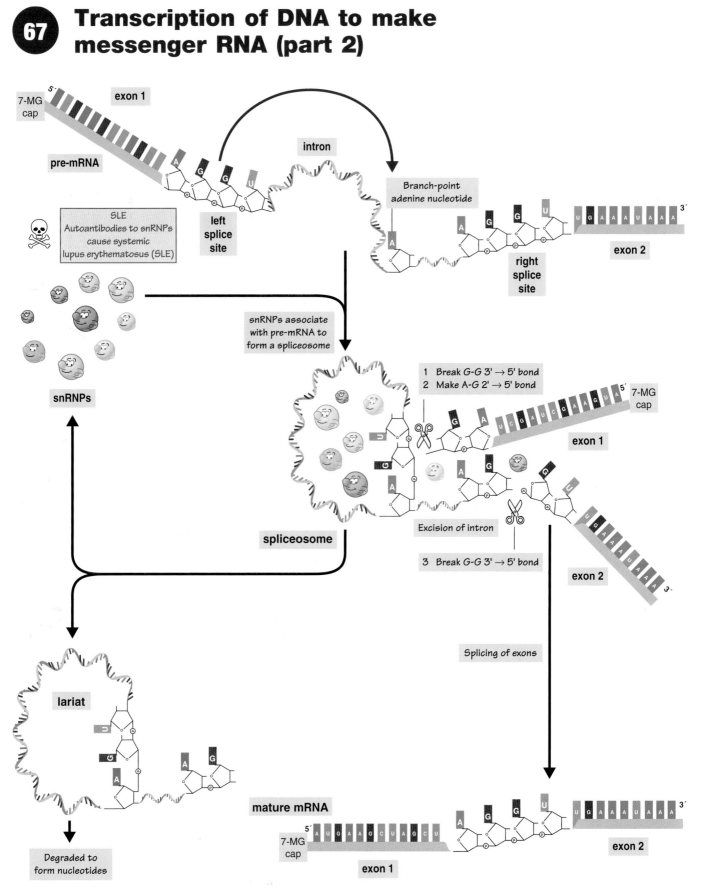

Figure 67.1 Processing of pre-mRNA in eukaryotes.

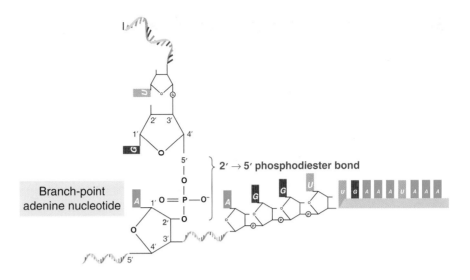

Figure 67.2 Detail of the 2′ → 5′ phosphodiester bond formed when an intron makes a lariat with the branch-point adenine nucleotide.

Branch-point
adenine nucleotide

2′ → 5′ phosphodiester bond

Pre-messenger RNA (pre-mRNA)

In the previous chapter (Chapter 66), we saw how in eukaryotes the first transcript of DNA by RNA polymerase II is **pre-mRNA**. This is composed of **exons** that contain the genetic information needed for protein synthesis. However, the exons are separated by non-coding lengths of DNA called **introns**. These are the remnants of gene building during evolution. Before the exons can be translated for protein synthesis, the introns must be removed and the remaining exons spliced together to make **mature mRNA**.

Pre-mRNA processing

The bases **AGGU** indicate the exon/intron borders and mark both the **left splice site** and the **right splice site**. This is possible because on the 5′ (left) border AG**GU** it is **GU** that marks the **left flank**. **Similarly**, on the 3′ (right) border **AG**GU, **AG** marks the **right flank**. From henceforth these will be described as "5′-AG**GU**" and "**AG**GU-3'" respectively.

Spliceosomes

Pre-mRNA processing is performed by a complex called the **spliceosome**. This is composed of small molecules of RNA known as **small nuclear RNA (snRNA)** and proteins to form several different types of **small nuclear ribonucleoprotein (snRNP**; usually pronounced "snurps"). One type of snRNP binds to the 5′ end (or left flank) of the intron while another type of snRNP binds to the 3′ end (or right flank) of the intron.

Branch-point adenine nucleotide

Within the intron is a specific **branch-point adenine nucleotide**. Several snRNPs bind to the intron causing it to loop so that the 5′-AG**GU**

border is adjacent to the branch-point adenine nucleotide (Fig. 67.2). The ribose–phosphate bond between G**G** is split, liberating exon 1, and the 5′-OH of **G** forms a 5′ → 2′ phosphodiester bond with the 2′-OH of the branch-point adenine nucelotide.

The lariat

Next the ribose–phosphate bond between **AG** is split, liberating exon 2, and the separated intron in the shape of a lariat is released and degraded to nucleotides.

Splicing of exon 1 to exon 2

Finally, the free 3′-OH of exon 1 reacts with the free 5′-phosphate of exon 2 to form a continuous length of mRNA ready for protein synthesis. NB In humans and other multicellular organisms, some pre-mRNAs can be spliced differentially in a controlled manner so that alternative exons can be used to make more than one mature mRNA, and hence more than one protein, from a particular gene. This capability enables the **human genome of 23,000 genes** to produce a **human proteome of 100,000 proteins**! For example, both **calcitonin** and the **neuropeptide calcitonin gene-related protein (CGRP)** originate from the same gene.

Systemic lupus erythematosus (SLE)

Patients with SLE produce autoantibodies against snRNPs and suffer the effects of aberrant pre-mRNA processing.

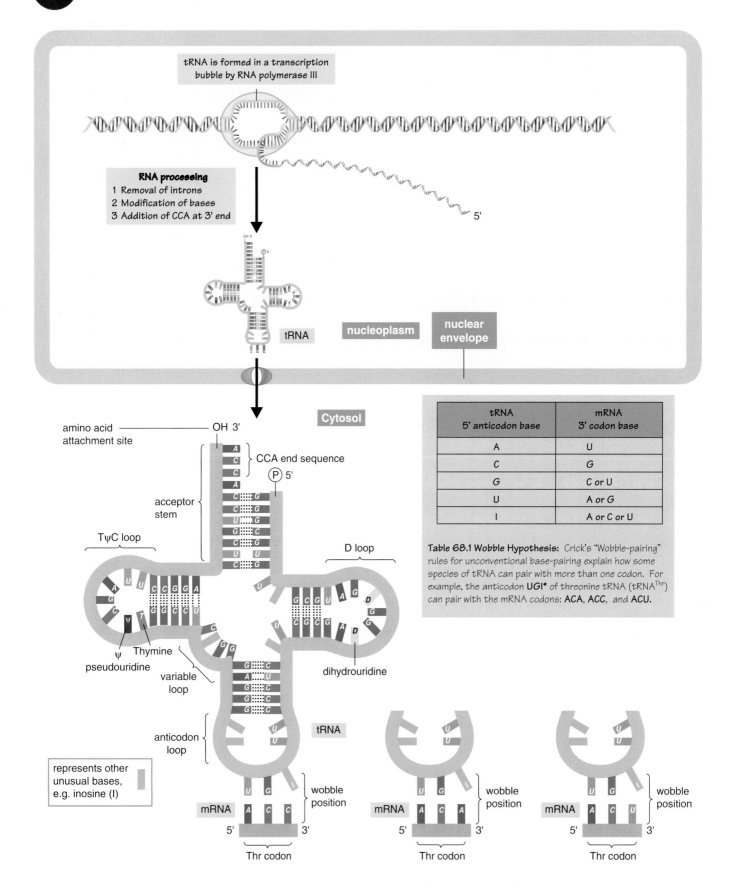

tRNA is formed in a transcription bubble by RNA polymerase III

RNA processing
1 Removal of introns
2 Modification of bases
3 Addition of CCA at 3' end

5'

OH 3'
P 5'

tRNA

nucleoplasm

nuclear envelope

amino acid attachment site

OH 3'

CCA end sequence

P 5'

A
C
C
A

acceptor stem

Cytosol

TψC loop

D loop

Thymine
ψ pseudouridine

variable loop

dihydrouridine

anticodon loop

tRNA

represents other unusual bases, e.g. inosine (I)

mRNA

5'   3'

wobble position

Thr codon

mRNA

5'   3'

wobble position

Thr codon

mRNA

5'   3'

wobble position

Thr codon

tRNA 5' anticodon base	mRNA 3' codon base
A	U
C	G
G	C or U
U	A or G
I	A or C or U

Table 68.1 Wobble Hypothesis: Crick's "Wobble-pairing" rules for unconventional base-pairing explain how some species of tRNA can pair with more than one codon. For example, the anticodon **UGI*** of threonine tRNA (tRNA^Thr) can pair with the mRNA codons: **ACA, ACC,** and **ACU.**

Synthesis of transfer RNA (tRNA) in eukaryotes and prokaryotes

In **eukaryotes**, the different types of tRNA are made by **RNA polymerase III** inside the nucleus (Fig. 68.1). The primary products of transcription undergo various modifications. All transcripts have a **C-C-A** group added to the 3′ hydroxyl end. Some precursors of tRNA have introns that are removed. Various bases are modified, forming unusual products (Fig. 58.2). For example, uracil can be altered to form **pseudouridine (ψ)** or reduced to form **dihydrouracil (D)**. Another example is **inosine (I)** formed by the deamination of adenosine.

In **prokaryotes**, all types of RNA, including the various types of tRNA, are made by **RNA polymerase**, which is a large complex composed of several subunits.

Structure of tRNA

Approximately 15% of the total RNA is transfer RNA. Each amino acid has at least one specific tRNA and the different types of tRNA contain from 75 to 95 nucleotides. Until recently tRNA was considered the smallest of the RNA family. However, since the mid-1990s a smaller type of RNA known as micro-RNA has been recognised (see below).

All tRNA molecules fold to form a stable, three-dimensional structure that when flattened resembles a clover leaf (Fig. 68.1). This is held together by hydrogen bonds according to base-pairing rules, resulting in looped, twisted and helical regions. All terminate at the 3′-hydroxyl end with the sequence **C-C-A**, which is the **amino acid attachment site**. Approximately 10% of tRNA consists of unusual bases. For example the **TψC loop** is characterised by **pseudouridine (ψ)** and **thymine bound to ribose** (not the usual deoxyribose). The **D loop** contains **dihydrouridine (D)**. The **variable loop** varies in size from 3 to 21 nucleotides. The four stems are rich in $G \equiv C$ base pairs providing **triple** hydrogen bond pairing, which gives structural stability. The **anticodon** end contains three bases that recognise the complementary **codon** triplets in mRNA. The example shown in Fig. 68.1 is **UGI**. This recognises three of the four mRNA codons for threonine: **ACA, ACC** and **ACU**. This is possible because of **tRNA wobble!**

Crick's tRNA wobble hypothesis

The genetic code comprises **four** different bases organised into codons comprising **three** of these bases. Thus 4^3 (i.e. **64**) **triplet codons** are possible in mRNA (Fig. 61.1). However, three of these mRNA triplets code "**STOP**". They bind to release factors (instead of tRNA) thereby terminating translation. This leaves **61 mRNA codons**. It might be assumed that 61 species of tRNA with 61 complementary anticodons are needed to pair with these codons, but this is not so. From the degeneracy seen in the genetic code (Table 61.1), Crick proposed "The Wobble Hypothesis" in 1966. He suggested that the first two bases of each codon formed perfect "Watson-Crick" pairings (A=U and G≡C) with the tRNA anticodon loop, but because of the constraints caused by the shape of the loop, the third base cannot get close enough. Model building suggested the pairing rules shown in Table 68.1 were responsible for codon-anticodon matching. This includes **inosine (I)** which was later discovered in the anticodon loop of some of the tRNA molecules.

Even with the "Wobble Hypothesis" more than 20 tRNA species are needed to cover the codons used by the 20 amino acids found in most proteins. *Escherichia coli* has 45 species of tRNA, from only one for phenylalanine or cysteine, to five for leucine.

Process of "charging" tRNA with amino acids: aminoacyl-tRNA synthetase enzymes

The function of the various tRNA molecules is to bind their specific amino acid. This is made possible by members of the **aminoacyl-tRNA synthetase family** of enzymes. These act as "match-makers" and are responsible for the accuracy of amino acid selection. They select their amino acid and marry it to its tRNA. First of all, the tRNA must be "charged" with its specific amino acid in a reaction catalysed by its specific aminoacyl-tRNA synthetase.

For example, **tyrosyl-tRNA synthetase** catalyses the reaction:

$$\text{Tyrosine} + \text{tRNA}^{\text{Tyr}} \xrightarrow[\textit{tyrosyl-tRNA synthetase}]{\text{ATP} \qquad \text{AMP} \;\; \text{PP}_i} \text{Tyrosyl-tRNA}^{\text{Tyr}}$$

Methionine is the exception. It can be attached to **two** types of tRNA depending on:

1 Whether it is acting in its special role as a **START** signal to initiate protein synthesis, i.e. "**initiator methionyl-tRNA**" (met-tRNA$_i^{\text{Met}}$) (Chapter 70).

2 If it is to be incorporated in the body of the protein like any other amino acid, i.e. just plain: "**methionyl-tRNA**" (met-tRNA^{Met}).

The charged tRNA then transfers its amino acid to the ribosome for incorporation into protein (Chapter 70). Here tRNA anticodons bind to a complementary codon on messenger RNA.

N-formylmethionine (fMet) in prokaryotes

fMet marks the starting point for prokaryotic protein synthesis and has a special transfer RNA, **tRNA^{fMet}**. Usually, **fMet** is removed from the completely formed protein.

Moonlighting enzymes

Recently, scientists at the Scripps Research Institute in the USA have discovered that human **tyrosyl-tRNA synthetase** does **two** jobs. In addition to its regular job in protein synthesis, i.e. charging tRNA^{Tyr} with tyrosine, it can also **stimulate** the growth of blood vessels. Also, another aminoacyl-tRNA synthetase, **tryptophanyl-tRNA synthetase**, not only charges tRNA^{Trp} with tryptophan, but it also **inhibits** the formation of new blood vessels. This research work has clinical potential. **Tyrosyl-tRNA synthetase** is **pro-angiogenic** and could be used to promote the growth of new blood vessels in some types of cardiovascular disease. On the other hand, **tryptophanyl-tRNA synthetase** is **anti-angiogenic** and could be used to reduce blood vessel invasion in cancer.

Micro-RNA (miRNA)

Traditionally tRNA has been acknowledged as the smallest member of the RNA family. However, recently an even smaller type of RNA, consisting of about 22 nucleotides, has been discovered. It is a family collectively called **micro-RNA (miRNA)**, members of which are thought to bind to their target mRNAs and control their stability.

Figure 68.1 Transcription of DNA to form tRNA. (NB 1. The base composition of the tRNA shown is stylised to represent a typical molecule of tRNA. 2. Anticodon **UGI***: by convention, sequences of both **codons** and **anticodons** are written from 5′ → 3′. Therefore, the anticodon in Fig. 68.1 when written is IGU: which is correct but confusing!)

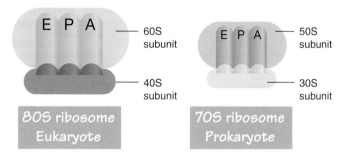

Figure 69.1 Eukaryote and prokaryote ribosomes.

Eukaryote ribosomes differ from prokaryotic ribosomes

Ribosomal RNA is the most abundant form of RNA and forms about 80% of the total. In combination with numerous proteins it forms the **ribosome** that is the work bench on which proteins are assembled from their constituent amino acids. The ribosome consists of two subunits. In **eukaryotes** a **40S** subunit combines with a **60S** subunit to form an **80S** ribosome (Fig. 69.1). **Prokaryotes** are different, they have a **30S** subunit that combines with a **50S** subunit to form a **70S** ribosome (Fig. 69.1).

Svedberg units: 40S and 60S refer to the sedimentation coefficients measured in Svedberg units "**S**". NB Sedimentation depends on the size and shape of macromolecules and so S units, unlike mass units, are **not** additive. For example, the 40S and 60S particles have molecular masses of 1.5 and 3.0 million g/mol, thus the intact ribosome has a mass of 4.5 million g/mol. However, the combined 40S and 60S particles combine to form a complete ribosome with a sedimentation coefficient of 80S.

E-site, P-site and A-site

Ribosomes (Fig. 69.1) contain three tRNA binding sites called **E-site**, **P-site** and **A-site** which are involved in protein synthesis (Chapter 70).

A-site. The **a**minoacyl, or **a**cceptor site binds the aminoacyl-tRNA which then transfers the aminoacyl group to the nascent polypeptide chain.

P-site. The **p**eptidyl site contains the tRNA bound to the polypeptide chain. *NB The initiating met-tRNA (or formylmet-tRNA in prokaryotes) binds to this site to start assembly of the ribosome and then polypeptide synthesis.*

E-site. The **e**xit site from which the **e**mpty tRNA leaves the ribosome.

Puromycin enters the A site, attaches to the polypeptide chain and then moves to the P site. The problem is it can neither accept the next aminoacyl group nor bind as it lacks the tRNA component: so polypeptide synthesis is terminated. Puromycin blocks both prokaryotic and eukaryotic protein synthesis. However, because diffusion into the eukaryotic cell is poor it is useful as an antibiotic in limited circumstances.

Biosynthesis of eukaryote ribosomal RNA

Biogenesis of ribosomes occurs in the nucleus where the rRNA genes are transcribed by **RNA polymerase I** to form **45S primary transcripts** (Fig. 69.2). The first 45S primary transcript functions as a **nucleolar organiser** and induces the formation of a **nucleolus** where multiple copies of the ribosomal RNA genes are transcribed into rRNA.

Now a series of processing events occur: the nascent pre-rRNA transcripts bind to proteins forming pre-ribonucleoprotein particles. A mature ribosome consists of approximately 67% RNA and 33% protein by weight. Spacers are excised from the 45S RNA releasing the **28S**, **5.8S** and **18S** rRNA components. The latter 18S rRNA with its associated proteins is diverted to form the **40S ribosomal subunit**.

Meanwhile, outside the nucleolus, the **5S** rRNA genes are transcribed by RNA **polymerase III**. The 5S rRNA produced moves into the nucleolus and associates with the 28S and 5.8S rRNA and various proteins to form the **60S ribosomal unit**. Both the 40S and 80S subunits migrate to the cytosol where, in combination with mRNA, they form **mature 80S ribosomes** during protein synthesis (Chapter 70).

The highly complex and stable folding of the rRNA molecules and their tight association with the various ribosomal proteins means that the ribosome subunits are extremely stable and can be used many times.

Prokaryote ribosomes

Since prokaryotes (by definition) have no nucleus, biogenesis of ribosomes occurs in the cytosol. Ribosomal RNA is made by a single multienzyme complex called **RNA polymerase**. Prokaryote ribosomes are much smaller than in eukaryotes. The large **50S subunit** is composed of many proteins plus **23S** rRNA and **5S** rRNA. The small **30S subunit** contains numerous proteins plus **16S** rRNA. The two subunits combine to form a **70S ribosome** (Fig. 69.1).

Although prokaryote ribosomes are very similar to eukaryote ribosomes, there are significant differences that are exploited by scientists working in the field of drug discovery. Compounds have been made that specifically target bacterial ribosomes inhibiting protein synthesis. For example, **tetracyclines** bind to the A site of the ribosome preventing aminoacyl-tRNA from attaching. They are used as a broad-spectrum bacteriostatic antibiotic.

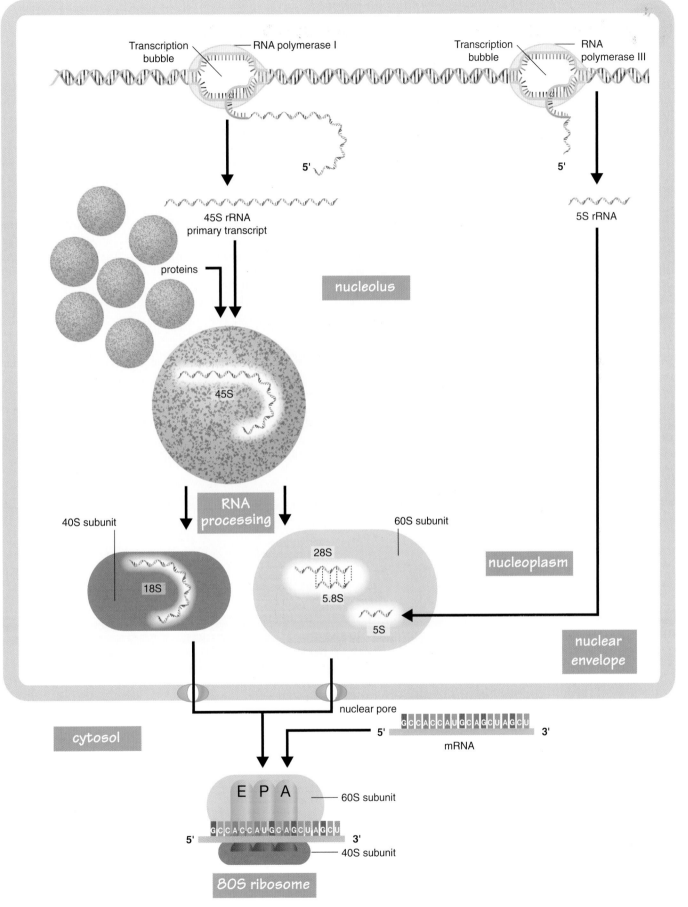

Figure 69.2 Biosynthesis of ribosomal RNA and formation of ribosomes in eukaryotes.

The genetic information coded in the sequence of base triplets in mRNA is **translated** to produce a sequence of amino acids, i.e. a protein in which the sequence of amino acids was predetermined by the genetic information. The process of translation and protein synthesis is summarised in Fig. 70.1 and in the following steps (of which steps 1 to 7 correspond to Fig. 70.1):

1 Charging tRNA with its amino acid. Amino acids are attached to their tRNA by a specific "match-maker" **aminoacyl-tRNA synthetase** (Chapter 68).

However, to initiate protein synthesis, a **special initiator** tRNA is needed: $tRNA_i^{Met}$. This reacts with methionine as shown in Fig. 70.1.

2 Initiation. Eukaryotic initiation factors (**eIFs**) are proteins that cooperate with *initiator* methionyl $tRNA_i^{Met}$. This binds to the **P site** of the **40S** ribosomal subunit complex, which now recognises the **7-methylguanosine cap** (**7-MG cap**) at the 5′ end of **mRNA**. The subunit scans along the mRNA until the **START** codon (**AUG**) is recognised.

3 Formation of the 80S initiation complex. Recognition of the **START** codon (**AUG**) in mRNA is assisted by the preceding "**Kozak sequence**" (Table 71.3) before the pre-initiation complex is formed. Finally, the **60S** ribosomal subunit combines with the **40S** subunit to form the **80S initiation complex**.

4 Elongation. The next aminoacyl-tRNA (in Fig. 70.1 it is **glycinyl-tRNA^{Gln}**) binds to the **A site** attracted by the next codon (**CAG**) of the mRNA. NB *Initiator* **methionyl-tRNA$_i^{Met}$** (the special one!) binds to the ribosomal **P site** whereas all other aminoacyl tRNAs bind to the

A site. The binding of the correctly charged tRNAs to the A site (as specified by the next mRNA codon) is assisted by the **elongation factors eEF1** and **eEF2** in eukaryotes. These also supply GTP, which provides the energy needed for protein synthesis.

5 Formation of the peptide bond. The two amino acids form a covalent peptide bond helped by the **peptidyl transferase** catalytic activity inherent in the ribosome 60S subunit (this "catalytic RNA" is known as a **ribozyme**).

6 and 7 Translocation and elongation. The ribosome now progresses three nucleotides towards the 3′ end of the mRNA locating the nascent peptide in the P site. Meanwhile, the initial tRNA, now empty of its amino acid, has moved to the **E site** where it exits the ribosome. The vacant **A site** is now free for the next aminoacyl-tRNA (which in Fig. 70.1 is **leucinyl-tRNA^{Leu}**).

8 Protein synthesis and termination. Reactions 4–7 are repeated one codon at a time and protein synthesis continues until a **STOP** codon is reached (**UGA**, **UAG** or **UAA**) when release factors (**RFs**) cooperate to liberate the completed protein.

9 Post-translational modification of protein. Often the initial protein that is synthesised is not functionally active. Chain-folding into a three-dimensional structure, modulated by "chaperone proteins", occurs during synthesis. However, for full functional activity, fine-tuning is usually needed after translation, e.g. de-methionation of the N-terminus, phosphorylation/dephosphorylation, glycosylation, disulphide bond reshuffling, relocation and aggregation with other proteins.

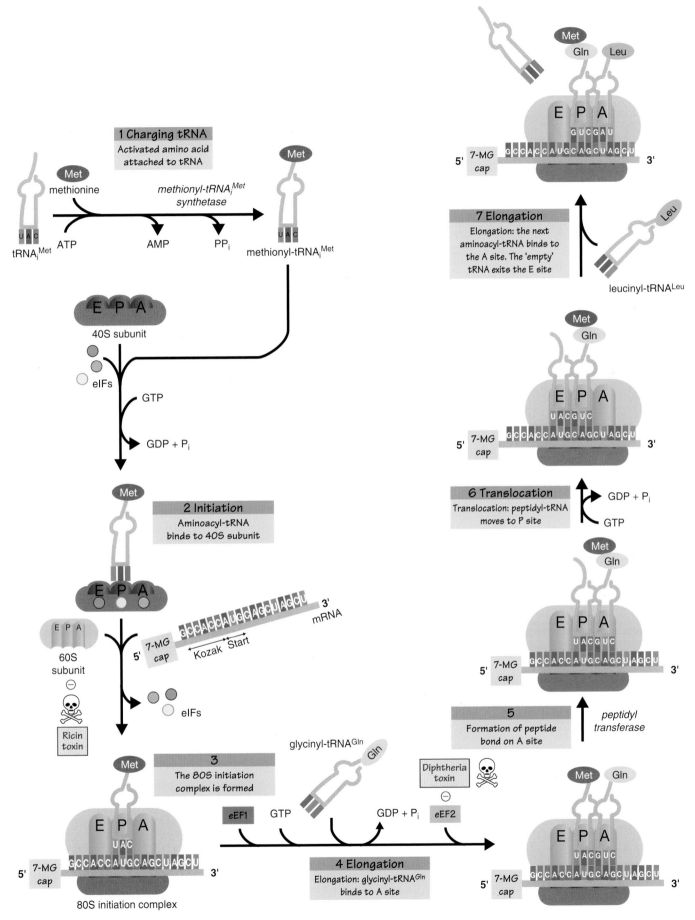

Figure 70.1 Translation of mRNA and protein synthesis in eukaryotes.

71 Comparison of DNA replication, DNA transcription and protein synthesis in eukaryotes and prokaryotes

Table 71.1 Summary and comparison of DNA replication in eukaryotes and prokaryotes (see Chapters 63 and 64). Numbers refer to Fig. 64.1.

	Process	Eukaryotes	Prokaryotes
	DNA structure	Linear DNA	Circular DNA
	Mechanism	**DNA replication is semiconservative**. Replication of the parent DNA produces two daughter DNA molecules; each of which consists of one parental strand and one daughter strand There is both **continuous** synthesis (**leading strand**) and **discontinuous** synthesis (**lagging strand** with **Okazaki** fragments)	
	Origin of replication	**Multiple** replication bubbles (Fig. 63.3)	**Single** replication bubble (Fig. 63.4)
1	DNA helicase and replication fork	DNA **helicase** unwinds the DNA double helix at the Y-shaped "**replication fork**"	
2	Single-stranded binding proteins	Keep the single strands apart at the replication fork preventing them from rejoining (reannealing)	
3	Super-coiling caused by helicase	**Gyrase** (prokaryotes) and **topoisomerase** (eukaryotes) cut and rejoin the DNA helix to relieve supercoiling	
		DNA topoisomerase: inhibited by anticancer drugs, e.g. etoposide	**DNA gyrase**: inhibited by antibacterial drugs, e.g. fluoroquinolones
4	RNA primer	**Leading** strand needs only **one** RNA primer. **Lagging strand** needs an RNA primer for **each Okazaki fragment**	
5	RNA primase	**DNA polymerase α** (also known as RNA primase) associates with DNA **polymerase δ**, forming a complex. **Primase** makes the **RNA primer** to which DNA is added by DNA polymerase δ	**Primase** makes the **RNA primer** to which DNA is added by **DNA polymerase III**

6	DNA polymerases	**Polymerase α**: also known as RNA primase (see step 5)
		Polymerase β: repairs DNA (Chapter 65)
		Polymerase δ: makes DNA on the lagging strand (Okazaki fragments)
		Polymerase ε: makes DNA on the leading strand
			1 **Polymerase III**: leading strand polymerase:
			  (a) **DNA polymerase**: extends the **leading strand**. Likewise for the **lagging strand** except it makes the **Okazaki fragment** up to the previously formed **RNA primer**
			  (b) **Proofreads** the new strand using 3′→5′ exonuclease activity
			2 **Polymerase I**: DNA repair enzyme, removes RNA primer:
			  (a) **RNase H activity**: 5′→3′exonuclease removes the RNA primer ("**H**" indicates that it acts on RNA/DNA "hybrid")
			  (b) **DNA polymerase activity**: fills the gap vacated by the RNA primer

7	Okazaki fragments	Approximately 100–200 deoxyribonucleotides	Approximately 1000–2000 deoxyribonucleotides
8	Removal of RNA primer leaves a "gap" that is filled with DNA	**Single primer** from the **leading** strand; **multiple primers** from the **lagging** strand removed by **RNase H** (RNase **H**: acts on a *hybrid* of RNA and DNA). **Polymerase δ** makes DNA to fill the gap vacated by the RNA primer	**Single primer** from the **leading** strand; **multiple primers** from the **lagging** strand removed by **polymerase I** which also makes DNA to fill the **gap** vacated by the RNA primer
9, 10	DNA ligase seals the "nick"	A **nick** remains at the 3′-hydroxy end of the Okazaki fragment. DNA ligase joins this 3′-hydroxy to the adjacent free 5′-phosphate group forming a phosphodiester bond	
11	Helicase and topoisomerase	Helicase and topoisomerase (eukaryotes) or gyrase (prokaryotes) advance along the DNA double-helix	
	Telomeres	**Telomerase**, an RNA-containing reverse transcriptase, adds "**TTAGGG**" repeats to the 5′ end of DNA forming a telomere which protects the end of chromosomes (Chapter 60)	Circular chromosomes. Circular DNA has no end, therefore has no need for telomeres!
	Fidelity of transcription (proofreading and editing)	During replication, errors occur in approximately one out of 10^{10} deoxyribonucleotides. Corrections (proofreading and editing) are made during the process of replication by the **3′→5′** exonuclease component of the DNA polymerase complex	

Table 71.2 Summary and comparison of DNA transcription in eukaryotes and prokaryotes (see Chapters 66–69).

Process	Eukaryotes	Prokaryotes
RNA polymerase	Different types of RNA polymerase: RNA polymerase II makes mRNA RNA polymerase III makes tRNA RNA polymerase I & III make rRNA	A single, multi-subunit complex makes mRNA, tRNA and rRNA
Promoter regions (switch on transcription)	Upstream promoter sequence CAAT followed by Core (or Basal) promoter TATA (Hogness box)	Sequence TTGACA (−35) followed by TATAAT (−10 or Pribnow box) are upstream of the transcription start (+1)
Enhancer regions	Sequences of DNA which enhance the rate of transcription	Not present in prokaryotes
mRNA Cap	5′-end protected by a 7-MG cap (7-methylguanosine cap)	Has a 5′-triphosphate cap. This is removed by phosphorylase enabling mRNA degradation to occur. mRNA has a half-life of a few minutes. Most mRNAs encode more than one gene product. In some cases, related enzymes in a pathway are transcribed as a single "poly-cistronic mRNA". Such clusters of functionally related genes are known as "operons", e.g. the lac operon. This gives coordinated control
mRNA Tail	mRNA has a poly-A tail	mRNA has a poly-A tail. Yes! Contrary to the popular belief stated in many textbooks, prokaryotic mRNA does have a poly-A Tail*

*Sarkar N. (1997) Polyadenylation of mRNA in prokaryotes. *Ann Rev Biochem* **66**, 173.

Table 71.3 Summary and comparison of protein synthesis in eukaryotes and prokaryotes (see Chapter 70).

Process	Eukaryotes	Prokaryotes
Ribosomal subunits	40S and 60S	30S and 50S
Ribosome complex	80S	70S
Protein initiation factors	Eukaryotic initiation factors (eIFs)	Initiation factors (IFs)
Start codon (AUG) codes for	Methionine	*N*-formylmethionine (fMet)
Initiation enhancing sequence upstream of start codon (AUG)	Kozak consensus sequence **GNCRCCAUG** (where **N** is any nucleotide and **R** is a purine)	Shine–Dalgarno consensus sequence AGGAGGNNNNNNNNNAUG (where **N** is any nucleotide)
Elongation factors	Eukaryotic elongation factors (eEFs)	Prokaryotic elongation factors (EFs)
Drugs/toxins	**Ricin** (toxin) from castor oil beans (*Ricinus communis*) is a ribonuclease that inhibits protein synthesis by cleaving and thus inactivating 28S rRNA. A single molecule of ricin within a cell attacks all the ribosomes and kills the cell **Diphtheria toxin**: an exotoxin secreted by *Corynebacterium diphtheriae* that inactivates eukaryotic elongation factor 2. A single molecule can kill a cell	**Aminoglycosides** prevent the formation of the initiation complex **Tetracyclines** bind to the A site and block the attachment of aminoacyl-tRNA **Chloramphenicol** inhibits peptidyl transferase (ribozyme) **Macrolides** and **clindamycin** bind to the 50S subunit and block translocation

72 Diagnostic clinical biochemistry (with Dr J. W. Wright FRCP, MRCPath)

NB [H+] indicates proton concentration which is inversely related to pH. (Chapter 1 & 2)

Measurement columns (reference ranges):

- Albumin (30–50 g/l or 3–6 g/dl)
- Calcium (2.0–2.5 mmol/l or 8–10 mg/dl)
- Phosphate (0.8–1.4 mmol/l or 2.5–4.3 mg/dl)
- Glucose Fasting < 6.0 mmol/l or < 108 mg/dl
- Creatinine (60–120 µmol/l or 0.6–1.3 mg/dl)
- Uric acid reference range – see below
- Urea (3–7 mmol/l or BUN 8–20 mg/dl)
- Bicarbonate (23–33 mmol/l)
- Potassium (3.5–5.0 mmol/l)
- Sodium (135–145 mmol/l)
- Total cholesterol (target <4.0 mmol/l or < 155mg/dl [for patients on treatment])
- Triglycerides (triacylglycerols) (< 1.5 mmol/l or < 133 mg/dl)
- Alkaline phosphatase Check local reference range
- Bilirubin (< 20 µmol/l or < 1.2 mg/dl)
- γ-Glutamyltransferase (γ-GT) Check local reference range
- ALT (alanine aminotransferase) Check local reference range
- LDH (lactate dehydrogenase) Check local reference range
- CK (creatine kinase) Check local reference range
- Free thyroxine (7–25 pmol/l or 0.5–2 ng/dl)
- TSH (thyroid-stimulating hormone) 0.3–5.0 mU/l

Other tests and comments

Kidney disease

Condition	Other tests and comments
Acute nephritis	Proteinuria, haematuria, casts, ASO titre ↑, complement ↓
Acute renal failure	Urinary Na ↓ in pre-renal failure
Chronic renal failure	If calcium is raised, possibility of primary tertiary hyperparathyroidism
Nephrotic syndrome	Heavy proteinuria. Differential protein clearance useful in assessing prognosis
Renal calculi	Check urine calcium, urate, oxalate. Rare possibility of cystinuria

Liver disease

Condition	Other tests and comments
Acute hepatitis	Check viral status (A, B and C), Urine bilirubin ↑ especially during recovery phase, occasionally anicteric. Check toxins
Acute hepatic necrosis	Prothrombin time prolonged. Bilirubin rises and enzymes fall as disease progresses
Chronic hepatitis: persistent	Check hep B antigen
Chronic hepatitis: active	IgG ↑, ANF and smooth muscle antibodies may be +ve
Primary biliary cirrhosis	Mitochondrial antibodies +ve, IgM↑, caeruloplasmin ↑
Portal cirrhosis	Prothrombin time prolonged, diffuse ↑ γ globulins, urinary urobilinogen ↑. Check for Wilson's disease (serum copper), haemochromatosis (serum iron), α-1-antitrypsin deficiency
Extrahepatic obstruction	Urinary bilirubin ↑
Infiltration/invasion	In localised liver disease, γ-GT and Alk Phos may be ↑ without jaundice
Haemolytic jaundice	Unconjugated bilirubin ↑, reticulocytes ↑, urinary bilirubin –ve, urinary urobilinogen ↑
Alcohol abuse	Consider measuring blood alcohol. MCV↑. NB Check for hypoglycaemia in alcohol coma especially in children

Cardiovascular disease

Condition	Other tests and comments
Myocardial infarction	Measure troponin I (or CK-MB) in acute situation. Sequence of enzyme elevation is: CK, AST, LDH
Cardiac failure	Raised enzymes may indicate ischaemic hepatitis

Gastrointestinal disease

Condition	Other tests and comments
Vomiting (with water replacement)	Dilutional hyponatraemia
Vomiting (without water replacement)	Changes are due to dehydration and chloride depletion
Bleeding	Urea is elevated especially in upper GI tract bleeding
Malabsorption	Faecal fat ↑, faecal elastase ↓. Folate, B12, and Ca may be ↓. Prothrombin time may be prolonged. Measure endomysial antibodies for celiac disease
Inflammatory bowel disease	May show some features of malabsorption
Diarrhoea	Changes are seen in prolonged diarrhoea
Acute pancreatitis	Serum amylase ↑ for 2–3 days. Serum methaemalbumin ↑ in severe cases

Respiratory disease

Disease	pO2 / pCO2 / pH notes
Acute respiratory failure	$pO_2 \downarrow$, $pCO_2 \uparrow$, $[H^+] \uparrow$, pH $\downarrow$ Uncompensated respiratory acidosis
Chronic respiratory failure	$pO_2 \downarrow$, $pCO_2 \uparrow$, $[H^+]$ N/$\uparrow$, pH N/$\downarrow$. Compensated respiratory acidosis

Bone and joint disease

- **Osteoporosis** Diagnosis depends on bone mineral density scan rather than biochemistry
- **Rickets & osteomalacia** Vitamin D $\downarrow$
- **Paget's disease** Calcium may increase with immobilisation
- **Primary hyperparathyroidism** PTH inappropriately high. Steroid suppression test: calcium remains high
- **Hypercalcaemia of malignancy** Steroid suppression test: calcium usually falls. PTH is not raised
- **Gout** Exclude renal dysfunction and diuretic treatment as cause of hyperuricaemia
- **Myeloma** Paraprotein band on electrophoresis. Confirm and characterise with immune electrophoresis; plasma cells $\uparrow$ in bone marrow, Bence-Jones proteinuria

Endocrine diseases

- **Diabetes mellitus** Diagnostic criteria: fasting blood glucose > 7 mmol/l and/or 2 hours post 75g glucose load > 11.1 mmol/l
- **Diabetic ketoacidosis** Glucosuria and ketonuria. Blood $[H^+] \uparrow$, pH $\downarrow$. Creatinine may be spuriously $\uparrow$ if measured by Jaffe method. NB Total body potassium and sodium are low
- **Hypothyroidism** TSH is used as first-line test for thyroid disorders
- **Hyperthyroidism** TSH unresponsive to TRH
- **Addison's disease (adrenal insufficiency)** Do synacthen test (if possible) before treating with steroids. Plasma cortisol $\downarrow$ and unresponsive to synacthen. Plasma ACTH $\uparrow$
- **Cushing's syndrome** Plasma and 24h urine cortisol $\uparrow$. Cortisol not suppressed by dexamethasone. Loss of diurnal variation of cortisol. Plasma ACTH inappropriately $\uparrow$ in pituitary Cushing's, very $\uparrow$ in ectopic ACTH, suppressed in adrenal Cushing's
- **Conn's syndrome** Plasma renin $\downarrow$, aldosterone $\uparrow$
- **Diabetes insipidus** Water deprivation test: polyuria persists; urine does not concentrate
- **Inappropriate ADH (SIADH)** Urine osmolality less than maximally dilute; urine sodium inappropriately $\uparrow$. Exclude adrenal insufficiency, renal failure and diuretic therapy

Sodium Large alterations are usually due to changed water balance. Often non-specifically $\downarrow$ in ill patients.

Potassium Spuriously elevated in unseparated or haemolysed specimens

Bicarbonate If the results are grossly abnormal check blood gases and $[H^+]$ (or pH)

Urea Increased in dehydration, but clinical signs are of more value. Varies with dietary protein

Uric acid Varies with dietary protein. Normal range: 0.12–0.42 mmol/l (male & post-menopausal female), 0.12–0.36 mmol/l (pre-menopausal female)

Creatinine Creatinine clearance usually gives no additional information

Glucose Timing with respect to meals is critical

Phosphate Falls after carbohydrate meals. Elevated in haemolysed/unseparated specimens

Calcium Total serum calcium related to albumin levels; adjusted by calculating "corrected calcium". Avoid venous stasis (falsely high values)

Albumin Many laboratory methods tend to overestimate low values

---

TSH Elevated in neonates (up to 40 mU/l)

Free thyroxine Non-specific decrease seen in many ill patients. Free T_3 also available

CK Originates from cardiac muscle, skeletal & smooth muscle and brain. Isoenzyme measurements used, particularly CK-MB in myocardial infarction

LDH Originates from liver, heart, skeletal muscle, red cells and kidney

ALT Moderately raised in obesity and metabolic syndrome. Marker for non-alcoholic fatty liver

γ-Glutamyltransferase (γ-GT) Increased with alcohol abuse and by other enzyme inducers, e.g. phenytoin, barbiturates and abdominal obesity

Bilirubin Gilbert's disease is a common cause of benign unconjugated hyperbilirubinaemia

Alkaline phosphatase Isoenzyme measurements may help to distinguish between bone, liver, intestinal and placental fractions. Raised during fracture healing, late pregnancy and in children during rapid growth

Triglycerides (triacylglycerols) Fasting specimen recommended

Cholesterol See British Joint Societies Lipid Guidelines (2004)

Legend:

- E$\downarrow$ — Epiphenomenon, low. Not of diagnostic value
- E$\uparrow$ — Epiphenomenon, high. Not of diagnostic value
- R$\uparrow$ — Rare, high. An uncommon association
- R$\downarrow$ — Rare, low. Not of diagnostic value
- ➡ — Tends to rise with progression of disease
- N — Normal
- N$\downarrow$ — Normal or low
- N$\uparrow$ — Normal or high
- $\uparrow$ — High to very high
- $\downarrow$ — Low to very low
- $\updownarrow$ — Low or high
- ⬇ Very low — Low
- ⬆ Very high — High

Index

abasic sites, 138
ABC (ATP-binding-cassette) motif, 90
ABC-A1, localisation, 90
ABCC8 gene, 57
acarbose, *48*
ACAT *see* acyl CoA–cholesterol–acyl transferase (ACAT)
ACE (angiotensin converting enzyme), *94*
acetaldehyde
    accumulation, *66*
    biosynthesis, 67
    metabolism, 67
acetaldehyde dehydrogenase, 67
    inhibition, *66*
acetate, biosynthesis, 67
acetic acid, 67
acetoacetate (AcAc), 65, *101*
    biosynthesis, 75
    proton production, 14
acetone, biosynthesis, 75
acetyl CoA, *51, 76*, 77
    biosynthesis, 31, *84, 85*
    metabolism, *84, 85*
    pyruvate dehydrogenase inhibition, 73
acetyl CoA carboxylase, *51, 120*
N-acetylneuraminic acid (NANA), 81
acid/base theory, 12–13
acidosis, 67
acids, 10–11
    definition, 10
    strong, 10
    weak, 10, 11, 14
    see also amino acids; carboxylic acids; fatty acids; α-ketoacids
acinar cells, proton production, 14
acne, 111
acquired immunodeficiency syndrome (AIDS), *126*
ACTH *see* adrenocorticotrophic hormone (ACTH)
acute hepatic necrosis, 152
acute hepatitis, 152
acute intermittent porphyria (AIP), *108*
    aetiology, 109
    symptoms, 109
    treatment, 109
acute nephritis, 152
acute pancreatitis, 152
acute renal failure, 152
acute respiratory failure, 153
acute tumour lysis syndrome (ATLS), *126*
    aetiology, 127
    treatment, 127
acyclic, definition, *46*
acyl carrier protein (ACP), components, *115*
acyl CoA–cholesterol–acyl transferase (ACAT), 92
    catalysis, 86
    inhibitors, 92
    storage, 86
acyl CoA dehydrogenases, *74, 115*
acyl CoA synthetase, *74*
ADA deficiency *see* adenosine deaminase (ADA) deficiency
Addison's disease, 153
    aetiology, 95
adenine, *26*, 28, 127, 128
    pairs, 128–9, 138
    structure, 125
adenine nucleotide, branch-point, *142*, 143
adenine phosphoribosyl transferase, 127
adenomas, 95
adenosine, 125, *126*
    deamination, 145
adenosine deaminase (ADA) deficiency, *126*
    aetiology, 127
adenosine diphosphate (ADP), *28, 35*
    accumulation, 29
    biosynthesis, 125

adenosine monophosphate (AMP), *28*, 73, 127
    accumulation, 53
    biosynthesis, 125
adenosine triphosphate (ATP), *50, 70*, 77
    biosynthesis, 100, 125
        aerobic, 28, 30–1
        anaerobic, 28–9, 73
        and insulin secretion, 57, *58*
        in muscles, *100*
        and ubiquinone, *84, 85*
        via anaerobic glycolysis, 42–5
        via fatty acid oxidation, 74–5
        via oxidative phosphorylation, 32–5, 36, 44
        yields, *40*, **42**, *74*
    demand, 71
    as energy, 40–1, 100–1
    functions, 28
    inhibitors, 33
    in mRNA synthesis, 140
    roles, 127
    structure, *28*
    struture, *125*
    as substrate, *71*
    turnover rate, 28
adenosine triphosphate synthetase, 31, 33, 36
    mechanisms, 32
    structure, 32
S-adenosylhomocysteine, *102*
S-adenosylmethionine (SAM)
    biosynthesis, *102*
    COMT reaction, *104*
    metabolism, 105
    and vitamin B₁₂, *118*
adenoviral vectors, 96
adenylate cyclase, activation, 58
adenylate kinase, catalysis, 28, 29
adenylate kinase reaction, adenosine triphosphate biosynthesis, 28–9
ADH *see* antidiuretic hormone (ADH)
adiponectin, 64
adipose tissue
    fatty acid esterification, 88, *89*, 92, *93*
    fatty acid mobilisation, *76*, 77
    fatty acid release, 65
    glycolysis, 73
    insulin activity, 95
    triacylglycerol storage, 50, *51*
    white, 77
ADP *see* adenosine diphosphate (ADP)
adrenal adenoma/carcinoma, 95
adrenal cortex, 95
adrenal glands, atrophy, 95
adrenal insufficiency, 153
adrenaline, *71*
    biosynthesis, 105
    catabolism, 105
    glycogenolysis stimulation, 58
    lipolysis stimulation, *76*
    metabolism, *104*, 105
    methylation, 105
    origin of term, 105
    overproduction, 105
    oxidative deamination, 105
    secretion, 105
adrenocortical insufficiency, aetiology, 95
adrenocorticotrophic hormone (ACTH)
    ectopic production, 95
    secretion, 95
advanced glycation end products (AGEs), 65
aerobic glycolysis, 73
aerobic oxidation, glucose, 40–1
agalsidase α, 81
ageing
    mechanisms, 33
    premature, 39
AGEs (advanced glycation end products), 65
aglets, 129
AIDS (acquired immunodeficiency syndrome), *126*

AIP *see* acute intermittent porphyria (AIP)
air hunger, 17
AKT
    and diabetes mellitus, *62*, 63
    signalling, 59
    use of term, 63
AKT gene, mutation, *62*, 63
5-ALA *see* 5-aminolevulinic acid (5-ALA)
δ-ALA *see* 5-aminolevulinic acid (5-ALA)
5-ALA synthase *see* 5-aminolevulinic acid (5-ALA) synthase
δ-ALA synthase *see* 5-aminolevulinic acid (5-ALA) synthase
alanine, *76, 97, 100*, 101, *106*
    biosynthesis, *98, 99*
    blood concentration, 31
    dissociation, 21
    pyruvate kinase inhibition in liver, *72*, 73
    structure, 20
    titration curve, *21*
    transamination, 96
alanine aminotransferase (ALT), 68, 116
    in serum, 152–3
    and vitamin B₆, *117*
β-alanine, *124, 125*
albinism, 105
    aetiology, 103
    oculocutaneous, 103
albumin, *76*, 77
    bilirubin binding, *109*
    glycated, 65
    in serum, 152–3
alcohol abuse, 67, 108, 114, 152
alcohol consumption, and fasting, 67
alcohol dehydrogenase, 66, 67, *70*
    roles, in ethanol metabolism, 67
alcohol metabolism, 66–7
alcoholism, *117*
    and thiamin deficiency, 73
aldolase A, *42, 44*
    deficiency, 45
aldolase B, 52
    deficiency, 53
aldose reductase, 49
aldoses, *47*
aldosterone, *16*, 85, 94–5
    biosynthesis, *94*
    deficiency, 95
aldosterone synthase, *94*
alkaline phosphatase, in serum, 152–3
alkaptonuria, *104*, 105
    aetiology, 103
allantoin, *126*, 127
allopurinol, *126*, 127
allosteric effectors, 71
ALT *see* alanine aminotransferase (ALT)
altitude, adaptation, 45
Alzheimer's disease, 23
Amadori product, *64*
Amanita phalloides (death cap mushroom), 141
α-amanitin, 141
amides, *20*
amines, methylated, 105
amino acid disorders, 102–3
amino acids, 20–1
    biosynthesis, 96, 148
    catabolism, 96–7
    classification, 20
    degradation, 100
    deletion, 22
    essential, 98–9
        catabolism, *99*
    glucogenic, 54, 101
    in gluconeogenesis, 65, 96
    hydrophobic R-groups, 20
    ketogenic, 54, 101
    metabolism, 100–1
        and vitamin B₆, *117*

nonessential, 98–9
    biosynthesis, 98, *117*
oxidation, 100, *114*, *115*
pH, 21
proton production, 14
R-groups, 21, 22
selection, in tRNA, 145
sequences, 131
solubility, *20*
structure, *20*, 21
tRNA attachment site, *144*, 145
tRNA charging, 145, 148, *149*
see also branched-chain amino acids (BCAAs)
amino groups, 21
    reactions, with glucose, *64*, 65
aminoacyl-tRNA, 148, *149*, **151**
aminoacyl-tRNA synthetases, 148, *149*
    functions, 145
aminoglycosides, **151**
β-aminoisobutyrate, *124*, 125
5-aminolevulinic acid (5-ALA), *108*
    accumulation, 109
    excretion, 109
5-aminolevulinic acid (5-ALA) synthase, *108*
    catalysis, 109
aminotransferases, catalysis, 97
ammonia, 30, 47, 125
    biosynthesis, 15, *17*
ammonium ions
    detoxification, *96*
    excretion, 15, *17*
    generation, 96, *97*
    metabolism, 96
    toxicity, 96
AMP *see* adenosine monophosphate (AMP)
α-amylase, *47*
amyloid proteins, 23
amyloidosis, 23
amylopectin, structure, *47*
amylose, structure, *47*
amytal, *32*, *33*, *34*
anabolic pathways, and NADPH, 27
anabolic steroids, *94*
anaemia
    chronic, 45
    haemolytic, 45, 112
    megaloblastic, 103, 119
    microcytic hypochromic, 109
    pernicious, *118*, 119
anaerobic glycolysis, 13, 42–5, *53*, 73
    proton production, 14
anaerobic oxidation, glucose, 42–3
anaesthetics, *19*
anastrozole, 95
androgenic alopecia, *94*, 95
androgens, 94–5
    biosynthesis, *94*
        impaired, 95
    precursors, 95
androstenedione
    biosynthesis, *94*
    as precursor, 95
angiotensin I, *94*
angiotensin II, *94*
angiotensinogen, *94*
α-anomers, of carbohydrates, *46*
β-anomers, of carbohydrates, *46*
anti-angiogenicity, tryptophanyl-tRNA synthetase,
    145
antibacterial drugs, **150**
antibiotics, *134*, 146
anticancer drugs, **150**
    delivery by liposomes, *82*
anticoagulants, 112
anticodons, *144*, 145
anticonvulsants, *108*
antidiuretic hormone (ADH), 153
    activity, 64
antifreeze, 67
antimetabolites, *122*, 125
antimycin A, *32*, *33*, *34*
antioxidants, 112
    measures, 39
antiparallel strands, 128
antipurines, mechanisms, 125

antipyrimidines, mechanisms, 125
antiseptics, 38
AP endonuclease, 138, *139*
AP sites, 138
apolipoproteins, *82*
    apoA1, *87*, *89*, *91*, *92*, *93*
        properties, **83**
    apoB48, *92*, *93*
        properties, **83**
    apoB100, 86, *87*, 88, *89*
        properties, **83**
    apoC2, *87*, 88, *89*, *91*, *92*, *93*
        properties, **83**
    apoE, *87*, 88, *89*, *92*, *93*
        properties, **83**
        removal, 86
    properties, **83**
apurinic sites, 138
apyrimidinic sites, 138
arachidonic acid, structure, *78*
5-ARD *see* 5α-reductase deficiency (5-ARD)
arginine, 29, 97, 101
    biosynthesis, 96, *99*
    catabolism, 99
    hydrolysis, 96
    as precursor, 96
    reabsorption disorder, 103
    structure, *20*
argininosuccinate, biosynthesis, 96, *97*
aromatase inhibitors, *94*, 95
arterial blood
    acidotic, 11
    alkalotic, 11
artichokes, Jerusalem, *46*
asbestos, 39
ascorbic acid *see* vitamin C
asparagine
    biosynthesis, 99
    structure, *20*
aspartate, 41, *97*, *100*, *101*, *117*
    biosynthesis, 98, 99
    in purine biosynthesis, *126*, 127
    in pyrimidine biosynthesis, *124*, 125
    reactions, with citrulline, 96
    structure, *20*
aspartate aminotransferase (AST), 96, *97*
astaxanthin, 110
atherosclerosis, 85, 86, *87*, 112
atherosclerotic plaque, *87*
athletes
    fuel consumption, 77
    nutritional supplements, 99
    performance enhancement, 29
    see also exercise
Atkin's Diet, 75
ATLS *see* acute tumour lysis syndrome (ATLS)
ATP *see* adenosine triphosphate (ATP)
ATP-binding-cassette (ABC) motif, 90
AUG, codon, 131, **151**
autoimmune diseases, 119
autophosphorylation, 58–9, 63
autosomal dominant inheritance, 64
autosomal recessive disorders, 81
avidin, *120*
azide, toxicity, 33

B-cells, 127
barbiturates, *108*
basal promoter, **151**
base excision repair, 138, *139*
base pairing, 128–9
    and hydrogen bonding, *128*
    rules, 137
bases, 10–11, 12
    amino acids, *20*
    definition, 10
    modification, in tRNA, *144*
    spontaneous deamination, and DNA damage,
        138
BBB (blood–brain barrier), 105
BCAAs *see* branched-chain amino acids (BCAAs)
beetle, *Trehala manna*, *47*
benign prostatic hypertrophy (BPH), 95
benserazide, *104*, 105
benzoate, *97*

beriberi
    dry, *114*
    wet, *114*
betaine, *102*, 103
BGP (bone Gla protein), 112
BH4 *see* tetrahydrobiopterin (BH4)
BHB *see* β-hydroxybutyrate (β-HB)
bicarbonate, *17*, 44
    biosynthesis, 14, 15
    buffer system, 11, 13, *17*
    increase, *19*
    overproduction, *16*
    in pyrimidine biosynthesis, *124*, 125
    reabsorption, 14, 15
    secretion, 14
    in serum, 152–3
bicarbonate ions, 96
bifunctional enzyme, deficiency, *44*, 45
bile, 85
bile salts
    biosynthesis, *84*, 85, 90
    enterohepatic circulation, *92*, *93*
    excretion, 86, *87*, 90, *91*
    reabsorption, 86
biliary obstruction, 111
bilirubin, 108–9
    binding, *109*
    biosynthesis, 109
    in serum, 152–3
bilirubin diglucuronide, biosynthesis, 109
biocytin, *120*
biotin, *51*, 77, *120*
    deficiency, *120*
    diagnostic tests, *120*
    dietary sources, *120*
    functions, *120*
biotin deficiency, non-dietary, *120*
biotinidase deficiency, *120*
bipolar disorder, mood changes, 107
birth defects, 110, 125
1,3-bisphosphoglycerate, *28*, *42*, 44
2,3-bisphosphoglycerate (2,3-BPG)
    and altitude adaptation, 45
    anaerobic glycolysis, 44–5
    biosynthesis, 44
    concentrations, 45
    in health and disease, 45
    metabolic effects, 45
    and smoking, 45
bisphosphoglycerate mutase
    deficiency, *44*, 45
    stimulation, *44*
2,3-bisphosphoglycerate phosphatase, deficiency, *44*, 45
2,3-bisphosphoglycerate shunt, 45
black pigments, 103
bladder, 103
bleach, 39
bleomycin, *122*
blood
    pH, *16*, *19*
    proton transport, 14–15
    see also arterial blood; red blood cells
blood–brain barrier (BBB), 105
blood calcium, 111
blood cholesterol, *79*
    lowering, 92
blood clotting
    mechanisms, 112
    times, 112
blood fatty acid concentration, 77
blood glucose concentration, *46*
    in diabetes mellitus, 55
    during fasting, 54, 55, 67, 77
    increase, 95
blood pressure, regulatory mechanisms, 39
blood proton concentration, regulatory mechanisms, 14
blood urea nitrogen (BUN), 152–3
Bohr effect, 44–5
α-1-bonding, carbohydrates, *47*
bonds, high-energy, 28
bone
    calcium resorption, 111
    metabolism, 112
    mineralisation, 112
bone Gla protein (BGP), 112

glucose 6-phosphatase, *60*
  deficiency, *61*
  localisation, 77
  nomenclature, *68*
  regulatory mechanisms, *58*
glucose 1-phosphate, *42*
  biosynthesis, 49, 58, 60
glucose 6-phosphate, *38, 42, 44, 51*
  accumulation, 50
  biosynthesis, 49, *72, 73, 76*
  metabolism, *50, 58*
glucose 6-phosphate dehydrogenase, deficiency, *38*
glucose 6-phosphogluconate, *38*
glucose toxicity, *46*
  mechanisms, 64–5
glucose transporters (GLUTs)
  GLUT2, *56–7, 60*
  GLUT4
    and glycolysis, 73
    translocation, *62, 63*
  GLUT5, fructose transport, 52
  roles, *72, 73*
glucose-dependent insulinotropic polypeptide (GIP), *56, 57*
D-glucose, *46*
α-D-glucose, *46*
β-D-glucose, *46*
α(1→4)-glucosidase, deficiency, *60*
α-glucosidase inhibitors, in type 2 diabetes treatment, *48*
glutamate, *76, 96, 97, 100, 101*
  biosynthesis, *17*, 96, *98, 99, 117*
  and malate/aspartate shuttle, *41*
  residues, 112
  structure, *20*
glutamate dehydrogenase, 15, *17*
glutaminase, 15, *17*
glutamine, *96*, 127
  biosynthesis, proton excretion, 15
  deamination, *17*
    proton excretion, 15
  in purine biosynthesis, *126*
  in pyrimidine biosynthesis, 125
  structure, *20*
glutamyl residues, 112
γ-glutamylcysteinylglycine (glutathione), *38*
γ-glutamyltransferase, in serum, 152–3
glutathione, oxidised, *38*
glutathione peroxidase, *38, 39*
glutathione reductase, 37, *115*
GLUTs *see* glucose transporters (GLUTs)
glycated plasma proteins, 65
glycated serum protein (GSP) *see* fructosamine
glycation, *46*, 55
  mechanisms, 64–5
  use of term, 65
glyceraldehyde, biosynthesis, 52
glyceraldehyde 3-phosphate, *42*
  biosynthesis, *44, 52*
glyceraldehyde 3-phosphate dehydrogenase, *40, 41, 44*
  catalysis, 42
glycerol, *82*
  biosynthesis, *74*
  and gluconeogenesis, 77
  mobilisation, 77
  structure, *78*
glycerol 3-phosphate
  biosynthesis, *41*
  fatty acid re-esterification, *51*
glycerol 3-phosphate dehydrogenase, 41
glycerol 3-phosphate shuttle, mechanisms, *40, 41*
glycine, *76, 100, 101*, 109, 127
  biosynthesis, *98, 99*
  in collagen, 24
  in purine biosynthesis, *126*
  structure, *20*
glycinyl-tRNA (tRNA ^Gln^), 148, *149*
glycoaldehyde, *67*
glycogen, *42, 48*
  abnormal accumulation, 60
  anaerobic oxidation, **42**
  as fuel reserve, 60
  liver, 54, 55, *60*
  structure, *46*
glycogen biosynthesis, 49, 50, 59, 62
  regulatory mechanisms, 58–9

glycogen metabolism, *117*
  regulatory mechanisms, 58–9, *71*
glycogen phosphorylase, *117*
  inhibition, 53
glycogen storage, 58, 60
glycogen storage diseases, and glycogenolysis, 60–1
glycogen synthase, *58*
  activation, 50, 59, 62, 63
  dephosphorylation, *71*
  inhibition, 59
glycogen synthase kinase-3 (GSK-3), *58, 59, 71*
  and diabetes mellitus, *62, 63*
glycogenesis, 50–1, 52
  mechanisms, *49*
glycogenin, *46*
glycogenolysis, 77
  and glycogen storage diseases, 60–1
  in health, 60
  inhibition, 53
  regulatory mechanisms, 58
glycolysis, 52, *115*
  aerobic, 73
  anaerobic, 42–5, *53*, 58, 73
    proton production, 14
  in cholesterol biosynthesis, 85
  functions, 73
  inhibition, *44*
  in liver, 73
  mechanisms, *40, 60*
  and pentose phosphate pathway, 49, 73
  reactions in, 28
  regulatory mechanisms, 72–3
  and vitamins, *114*
glycolytic enzymes, deficiency, 45
glycoproteins, 24, *82*
  biosynthesis, 85
glycosylation, use of term, 65
Glyset, *48*
gout, *61, 126*, 153
  aetiology, 127
  treatment, 127
GSH (glutathione), *38*
GSK-3 *see* glycogen synthase kinase-3 (GSK-3)
GSP *see* fructosamine
GSSG (oxidised glutathione), *38*
GTP *see* guanosine triphosphate (GTP)
guanine, *126*, 128
  oxidation, 138
  pairs, 128–9
  structure, 125
guanosine, 125, *126*
guanosine caps, 140
guanosine triphosphate (GTP), 77
  biosynthesis, *28*
  in mRNA synthesis, 140
  roles, 127
guardian angel protein, 123
Guillain–Barré syndrome, and respiratory acidosis, *19*
Günther's disease, aetiology, *108*
gyrase, 137, **150**

Haber–Weiss reaction, *38, 39*
haem
  biosynthesis, 109
  catabolism, 109
  metabolism, 108–9
  proteins, 109
haem oxygenase, catalysis, 109
haemarginate, *108*
haematin, *108*, 109
Haematococcus pluvialis (alga), 110
haemin, *108*
haemoglobin, *108*
  biosynthesis, 65, 109
  oxygen release, 44
  and plasma glucose concentration, **65**
  structure, 45
  see also deoxyhaemoglobin; fetal haemoglobin
haemoglobin A$_{1c}$
  biosynthesis, 65
  classification, 65
haemolysis, 113
haemolytic anaemia, 45, 112
haemolytic jaundice, 152
haemopoietic stem cells, 81, 109

haemopoietic tissue, 119
haemorrhage, neonatal, 113
haemorrhagic disease of the newborn, 113
β-HB *see* β-hydroxybutyrate (β-HB)
HbA$_{1c}$ *see* haemoglobin A$_{1c}$
25-HCC (25-hydroxycholecalciferol), 111
HCO$_3^-$ *see* bicarbonate
HCU *see* homocystinuria (HCU)
HDL (high density lipoprotein) receptors, *91*
HDLs *see* high density lipoproteins (HDLs)
heart attack *see* myocardial infarction
heart disease
  congenital, 45
  see also cardiovascular disease
Helianthus tuberosus (Jerusalem artichoke), inulin, *46*
helicase, *136*, 137, **150**
α-helices, 24
  right-handed, 22, *23*
Henderson-Hasselbalch equation, 11
hep C, *108*
hepatic failure, *18, 47*
hepatic fructokinase deficiency, 52, *53*
hepatic nuclear factor 1 alpha (HNF1A), 57, 64
hepatic nuclear factor 1 beta (HNF1B), 64
hepatic nuclear factor 4 alpha (HNF4A), 64
hepatic portal vein, 49, 73, 86, 88
  bile salt absorption, 90, *93*
hepatitis, 152–3
hepatomegaly, *61, 108*
hereditary fructose intolerance (HFI)
  aetiology, 53
  pathology, 53
  treatment, 53
hereditary non-polyposis colorectal cancer (HNPCC), 138
heterochromatin, 132–3
  structure, *133*
heterogeneity, 31
heteroplasmy, 31
hexadecanoate *see* palmitate
hexadecanoic acid *see* palmitic acid
hexokinase, *40, 42, 44, 70, 73*
  catalysis, *50, 52*
  deficiency, 45
  glucose affinity, 73
  and glycolysis regulation, 73
  occurrence, 73
β-hexosaminidase A, deficiency, *81*
hexose monophosphate shunt pathway *see* pentose phosphate pathway
HFI *see* hereditary fructose intolerance (HFI)
HI *see* hyperinsulinism (HI)
5-HIAA (5-hydroxyindoleacetic acid), *106, 107*
high density lipoprotein (HDL) receptors, *91*
high density lipoproteins (HDLs), *79, 82*, 88
  cholesterol transport, *84*, 92
  functions, 90
  metabolism, reverse cholesterol transport, 90–1
  properties, **83**
  roles, 85
hippurate, 97
hirsuitism, *94*
histamine, 107
histidine, *76, 98, 100, 101*
  catabolism, 99
  metabolism, products, 106–7
  one-carbon transfer, 119
  structure, *20*
histones, *133*, 137
HIV (human immunodeficiency virus), 131
HMGCoA (3-hydroxy-3-methylglutaryl CoA), *84, 85*
HMGCoA reductase *see* 3-hydroxy-3-methylglutaryl CoA (HMGCoA) reductase
HMMA (4-hydroxy-3-methoxymandelate), *104, 105*
HNF1A (hepatic nuclear factor 1 alpha), 57, 64
HNF1B (hepatic nuclear factor 1 beta), 64
HNF4A (hepatic nuclear factor 4 alpha), 64
HNPCC (hereditary non-polyposis colorectal cancer), 138
Hogness box, 140, **151**
homocysteinaemia, aetiology, 119
homocysteine, *117*
  accumulation, 103
    blood concentration, 102
    serum concentration, 103

RNA, *47*
    bases, *124*, 125
    biosynthesis, 127
        and vitamins, 119
    see also mRNA; snRNA
RNA polymerase, 140, 145, **151**
RNA polymerase I, 141, 146, *147*, **151**
RNA polymerase II, 140, 141, **151**
RNA polymerase III, 141, *144*, 145, *147*, **151**
RNA primase, *134*, *136*, 137, **150**
RNA primers, *136*, 137, **150**
RNA processing, *144*
    rRNA, *147*
RNA viruses, 131
RNase H, **150**
ROS *see* reactive oxygen species (ROS)
rotenone, *32*, *34*
    pesticidal activity, 33
    toxicity, 33
rRNA, *130*, 131
    abundance, 146
    biosynthesis
        eukaryotes, 146, *147*, **151**
        prokaryotes, 146, **151**
        via DNA transcription, 146–7
    inactivation, **151**

salicylates, *18*
salvage pathway, 125
    purine, 127
    pyrimidine, *124*, 125
    see also methionine salvage pathway
SAM *see* S-adenosylmethionine (SAM)
sarcoidosis, vitamin D hypersensitivity, 111
sarcomas, 111
Schiff bases, *64*
Schilling test, 119
SCID *see* severe combined immunodeficiency (SCID)
scrapie, 22–3, 131
scurvy, *24*, *25*
    aetiology, *121*
seafood, 110
Selaginella lepidophylla (Resurrection plant), *47*
selective serotonin re-uptake inhibitors (SSRIs), 106
selenium-dependent enzymes, 39
self-mutilation, 127
semiquinones, 39
sepsis, *18*
serine, *76*, 80, 81, *100*, 101
    biosynthesis, *98*, 99
    genetic coding, **131**
    one-carbon transfer, 119
    phosphorylation, *63*, *71*
    structure, *20*, *80*
serotonin
    biosynthesis, 106
    deficiency, and depression, 106, 107
severe combined immunodeficiency (SCID), *126*
    aetiology, 127
sex hormones, 95
sex steroids, porphyria, *108*
sexual characteristics, secondary, *94*
β-sheets, 24
    antiparallel, *22*
    parallel, *22*
Shine–Dalgarno consensus sequence, **151**
SIADH (syndrome of inappropriate antidiuretic hormone
        secretion), 153
sialic acid (*N*-acetylneuraminic acid), 81
signal transduction, insulin, *62*–3
signalling proteins, *58*–9
silencers, 140
single replication bubbles, 135, **150**
single-stranded binding proteins (SSBs), *134*, *136*, 137
single-stranded DNA (ssDNA), 132
singlet oxygen, *38*
    biosynthesis, in porphyria, *108*, 109
    neutralisation, 110
skeletal muscle, 73
    fuels, 99
    glycogenolysis, *60*
    phosphorylase deficiency, *61*
skin cancer, 103, 138
SLE (systemic lupus erythematosus), *142*, 143

slimming pill, DNP claims and toxicity, 36
small cell lung carcinoma, 95
small nuclear ribonucleoprotein (snRNP), *142*, 143
small nuclear RNA (snRNA) *see* snRNA
smoking
    and 2,3-bisphosphoglycerate levels, 45
    and lung damage, 39
snRNA, 143
snRNP (small nuclear ribonucleoprotein), *142*, 143
SOD *see* superoxide dismutase (SOD)
sodium, in serum, 152–3
sodium calcium edetate, *108*
sodium ions, aldosterone, *94*
solenoids, chromatin structure, *133*
sorbitol, structure, *47*
sphingolipidoses, degradation, *81*
sphingolipids, 80–1
    degradation, *81*
    properties, *81*
    structure, *80*
sphingomyelin
    biosynthesis, 81
    structure, *80*
sphingomyelinase, deficiency, *81*
sphingosine
    biosynthesis, 81
    structure, *80*
spina bifida, 119
spinal cord, and respiratory acidosis, *19*
spindle fibres, *122*
splenomegaly, *108*
spliceosomes, *142*, 143
spongiform encephalopathies, aetiology, 22–3
spontaneous deamination of bases, and DNA damage,
        138, *139*
squalene, *84*
SREBP-2 *see* sterol responsive element binding
        protein-2 (SREBP-2)
SSBs (single-stranded binding proteins), *136*, 137
ssDNA (single-stranded DNA), 132
SSRIs (selective serotonin re-uptake inhibitors), 106
stanols, 92
Staphylococci spp., and chronic granulomatous disease,
        37
starch
    digestion, *47*, *48*, 50
    structure, *47*
start codon, 145, 148, *149*
starvation
    blood glucose concentration, 77
    brain fuel requirement during, 54
    and gluconeogenesis, *76*, 77
    and glycogen mobilisation, 60
    phases, *54*, 55
    see also fasting
statins, *84*, 85, *86*
    and ubiquinone, 85
stearic acid, 79
    structure, *78*
steatorrhoea, 110, 112
    and vitamin D, 111
steatosis, 50
    and alcohol metabolism, 66–7
stem cells, haemopoietic, 81, 109
stercobilin, biosynthesis, 109
steroid hormones, 94–5
    biosynthesis, *94*
    precursors, 85
    types of, 95
steroids, and depression, 107
sterol responsive element binding protein-2 (SREBP-2),
        87, *93*
    roles, *70*
sterols, in margarines, 92
stop codons, 131, 145, 148, *149*
β-strands, *22*, 24
stroke, and respiratory acidosis, *19*
succinate, *31*, *32*
    biosynthesis, *28*
succinate dehydrogenase, *31*, *32*, 32, *40*, 74, *115*
succinyl CoA, *108*, 109
    biosynthesis, *100*, *101*
succinyl CoA synthetase, *28*, 28, *40*, 74
sucralose, sweetener, *48*

sucrase deficiency, *48*
sucrase/isomaltase, 52
    deficiency, *48*
sucrose, *47*, 50
    absorption, *48*
    hydrolysis, 52
    occurrence, *48*
    structure, *48*
sudden infant death syndrome (SIDS), biotin and
        aetiology, 120
sugar alcohols, *47*
sulphonamides, porphyria, *108*
sulphonylurea receptor 1 (SUR1), *56*–7
    mutation, 57
sulphonylureas, *56*, 57
sulphur, binding, *70*
sulphydryl group, *26*
sunflower oil, 79
sunlight, lack of, 111
super-coiling, **150**
superoxide anion radicals, 36–7
    biosynthesis, 39
superoxide anions, *38*, 39
superoxide dismutase (SOD), 37
    defence mechanisms, *38*, 39
SUR1 *see* sulphonylurea receptor 1 (SUR1)
Svedberg units, 146
sweeteners, *47*, *48*
synapses, 107
synaptotagmin, *56*
syndrome of inappropriate antidiuretic hormone
        secretion (SIADH), 153
systemic lupus erythematosus (SLE), *142*, 143

T-cells, 127
T1DM *see* type 1 diabetes (T1DM)
T2DM *see* type 2 diabetes (T2DM)
TAGs *see* triacylglycerols (TAGs)
TATA box, 140, **151**
taxols, *122*
Tay-Sachs disease, *81*
telomerase, 129, **150**
telomeres, 129, *132*, *133*, **150**
tendon xanthomata, 85
termination, of transcription, 140
testosterone, 85, *94*, 95
testosterone receptor blockers, 95
tetany, 111
tetracyclines, **151**
tetrahydrobiopterin (BH4)
    as co-factor, 105
    loading test, 105
tetrahydrobiopterin-responsive phenylketonuria, 105
tetrahydrofolate (THF), 119, 127
    biosynthesis, 125
tetramers, 24
B⁺-thalassaemia, 141
thermogenesis
    non-shivering, 36
    and proton leakage, 36
thermogenin *see* uncoupling protein 1 (UCP1)
THF *see* tetrahydrofolate (THF)
thiamin, *26*, 31, *72*
    deficiency, 73
    do not confuse with thymidine, 125
    see also vitamin B₁
thiamin pyrophosphate (TPP) *see* vitamin B₁
thiazide diuretics, *16*
threonine, *100*, 101
    catabolism, 99
    phosphorylation, *63*, *71*
    structure, *20*
    tRNA, 145
threonine tRNA (tRNA^Thr), *144*
thymidine, 125
thymidylate synthase, *124*
    inhibition, 125
thymine, *124*, 128, *144*
    bound to ribose in tRNA, 145
    dimerisation, 138, *139*
    pairs, 128–9
    structure, 125
thymocytes, 127
thyroid stimulating hormone (TSH), in serum, 152–3

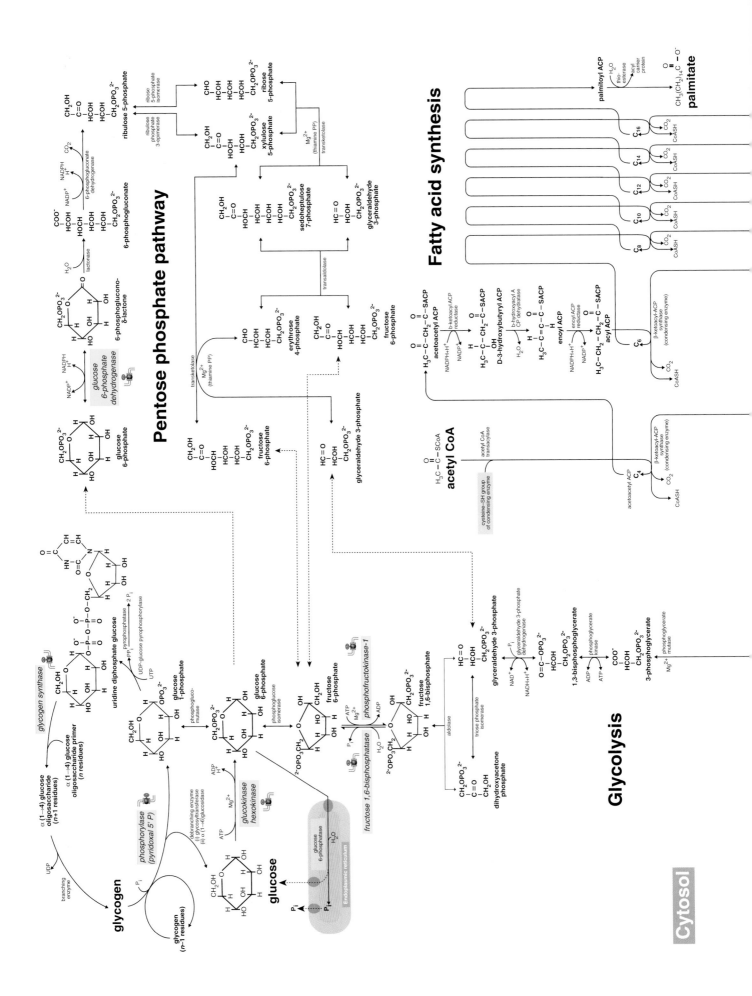

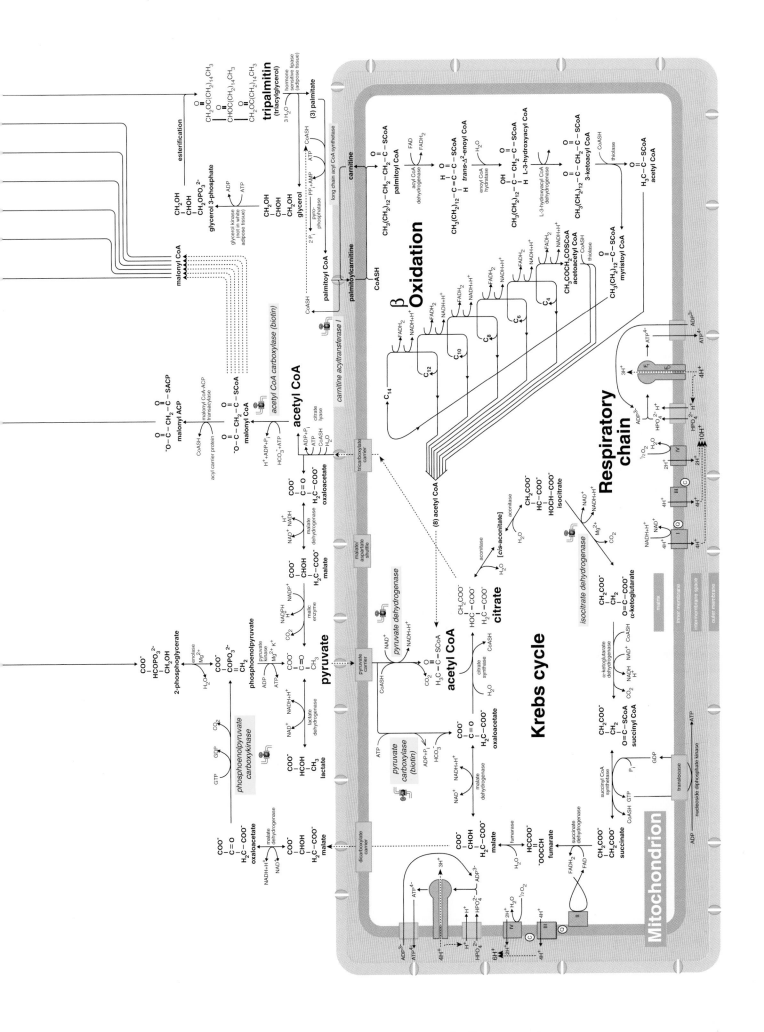